The Keto Vegetarian

84 Delicious Low-Carb Plant-Based,
Egg & Dairy Recipes for A Ketogenic Diet
(Nutrition Guide)

The Carbless Cook 1
By Lydia Miller
Version 2.1
Published by **veganvegetarianketo**

D1473413

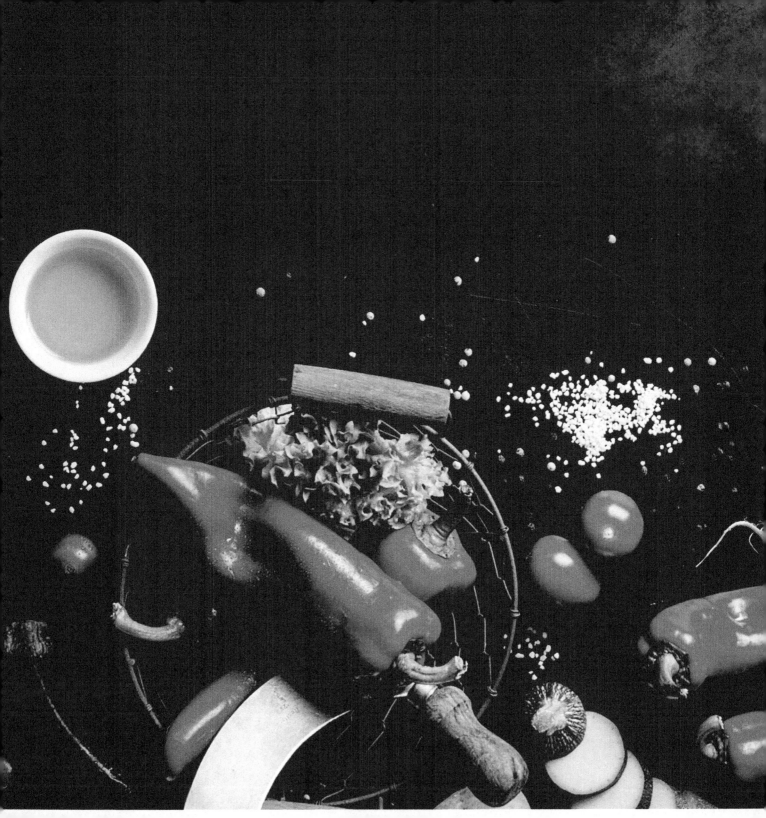

Introduction

Ketogenic and vegetarian diets have gained a lot of attention in recent years as a result of unprecedented chronic illness epidemics and a general shift toward a health-conscious way of life, as well as growing humanitarian and environmental concerns. This book will serve as a guide to the low-carbohydrate high-fat (LCHF) vegetarian diet, providing both background information and a range of recipes, which will aid the successful adoption of the diet.

The ketogenic vegetarian diet is exactly what is sounds like. It combines the ketogenic diet with the vegetarian diet. Vegetarians do not consume meat or fish, but unlike vegans, other animal products are permitted. Many people choose to adopt this lifestyle for religious, moral, and/or health reasons.

There has been a lot of controversy surrounding the adoption of plant-based diets, and many people still believe that such diets are detrimental to one's health. Over the past 30 years, however, evidence has increasingly suggested that (mostly) plant-based diets are actually healthier than traditional western diets in which meat consumption is high, which results in high intake of saturated fat, cholesterol, calories, carcinogenic preservatives, salt, sugar, and chemical byproducts from the cooking process[i]. Guidelines have been established for those who wish to be able to successfully adopt plant-based diets in a healthy and responsible way. These include ensuring adequate intake of plant foods high in iron and protein, as well as supplementation[ii] of some micronutrients such as vitamin B12.

The ketogenic diet, on the other hand, is based on the reduction of blood glucose through the restrictive consumption of carbohydrates, the energy source from which glucose is derived. Glucose typically serves as the body's main source of fuel so doing this results in the production of alternative energy sources by the liver's ketone bodies – a source of energy produced from the breakdown of stored fats. Studies have shown that the short-term effects of the ketogenic diet are weight loss, reductions of low-density lipoproteins (LDL), and blood triglycerides, which all lower the risk of cardiovascular diseases.

The vegetarian ketogenic diet allows for the consumption of both plant fats, such as the fats found in vegetable oils, nuts, seeds, avocados, and animal fats, found in dairy and eggs. Therefore, the vegetarian ketogenic diet allows for a lot of variety and nutritional freedom while mitigating the harmful bodily, environmental, and moral consequences of meat and fish consumption.

The possibility of being able to improve your health while contributing to the betterment of the world, not to mention continuing to enjoy delicious food may seem too good to be true. With the help of this book, you will see how simple it is to accomplish this. Innocent animal lives and your health do not have to be sacrificed for good-tasting food. As you read through these lessons, you will find yourself letting go of outdated and questionable beliefs and embracing a new low-carb, guilt-free lifestyle!

Disclaimer

The recipes provided in this report are for informational purposes only and are not intended to provide dietary advice. A medical practitioner should be consulted before making any changes in your diet. Additionally, recipe cooking times may require adjustment depending on age and quality of appliances. Readers are strongly urged to take all precautions to ensure ingredients are fully cooked in order to avoid the dangers of foodborne viruses. The recipes and suggestions provided in this book are solely the opinion of the author. The author and publisher do not take any responsibility for any consequences that may result due to following the instructions provided in this book.

Congratulations with your responsible and health-conscious decision to read my book.

I'm very excited for you!

I offer my readers an exclusive opportunity to become part of my keto circle. Dozens of people are already inside and enjoying *extra* (vegan & vegetarian) ketogenic recipes and support on their journey to fat-fueled cooking, more energy and weight loss.

Join a growing number of 'plant-ketoers' and become part of my circle today at

http://tiny.cc/ketocircle!

You'll get '*The Keto Vegetarian: 8 Reader-Exclusive Low-Carb, Plant-Based, Egg & Dairy Recipes*' as a welcome gift!

Subscribe to my newsletter and join dozens of people with similar goals (and ethics) here:

http://tiny.cc/ketocircle!

(I absolutely hate spam and will never email you more than twice a week.)

As a member of my keto circle, you will receive some of my latest recipes, exclusive opportunities to get new releases free of charge, and more...!

As a member of my keto circle, you can also always reach out for personal questions!

My Facebook page: **https://www.facebook.com/veganvegetarianketo** is also great to stay up-to-date and reach out.

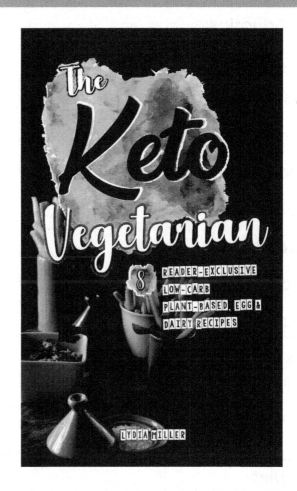

Our Facebook group: **https://www.facebook.com/groups/veganvegetarianketo** is where you get inspired, can share results directly with other 'plant-ketoers' and stay motivated on your keto journey!

See you inside!

Lydia

Table of Contents

What is the Ketogenic Diet?

The typical proportional intake of macronutrients is around 45-65% carbohydrates, 20-35% fats, and 15-20% proteins. Carbohydrates are broken down more easily, which is why they serve as the body's primary source of fuel for immediate energy supply. Fat, on the other hand, is broken down less efficiently, so it is typically stored as an alternative fuel source for when glucose is not readily available. Proteins are used primarily for structural functions such as tissue repair and enzyme production and are only used as a source of fuel in a state of starvation.

In order to understand ketosis, it is important to understand the role of glucose beyond its function as an immediate source of energy derived from the digestion of carbohydrates. The body also converts excess glucose to glycogen, a long-term energy storage found in the liver and the muscles. Under caloric restriction, glycogen is converted back into glucose to keep glucose levels in the blood within the normal range. In muscle tissue, it is broken down on-site to provide energy for muscle activity.

If glycogen stores are depleted, the body will rely on protein and fat from the diet for energy. Most cell types are able to use fatty acids as a fuel source. Fat stores will also be broken down, leading to weight loss.

In order to induce the breakdown of fat, which goes hand in hand with ketosis, fewer carbs and more fat need to be consumed, and carbohydrates should be complex, as these require more energy to be broken down and produce a more gradual release of glucose into the blood. Complex carbs are found in ingredients such as veggies, whole grains, beans, and lentils. On a strict ketogenic regime, protein is also restricted because it triggers the release of a growth factor that stimulates the uptake of glucose from the blood.

As fatty acids are mobilized from adipose tissue (fat stores), the ketogenic pathway is activated in the liver, converting acetyl-CoA into ketone bodies, which are then used as fuel. Ketone bodies represent three water-soluble molecules: beta-hydroxybutyrate, acetoacetate, and acetone.

Ketogenic diets are effective in the short-term for weight loss and treatment of cardiovascular risk factors. Long-term, a more moderate diet such as a low-carb diet can be adopted in order to make it sustainable and avoid muscle loss. It is crucial that the ketogenic diet is carried out correctly. Failure to do so can result in illness or other serious health problems. Long-term ketogenic diets prescribed by a dietician or doctor for medical reasons should be followed strictly according to his/her guidelines.

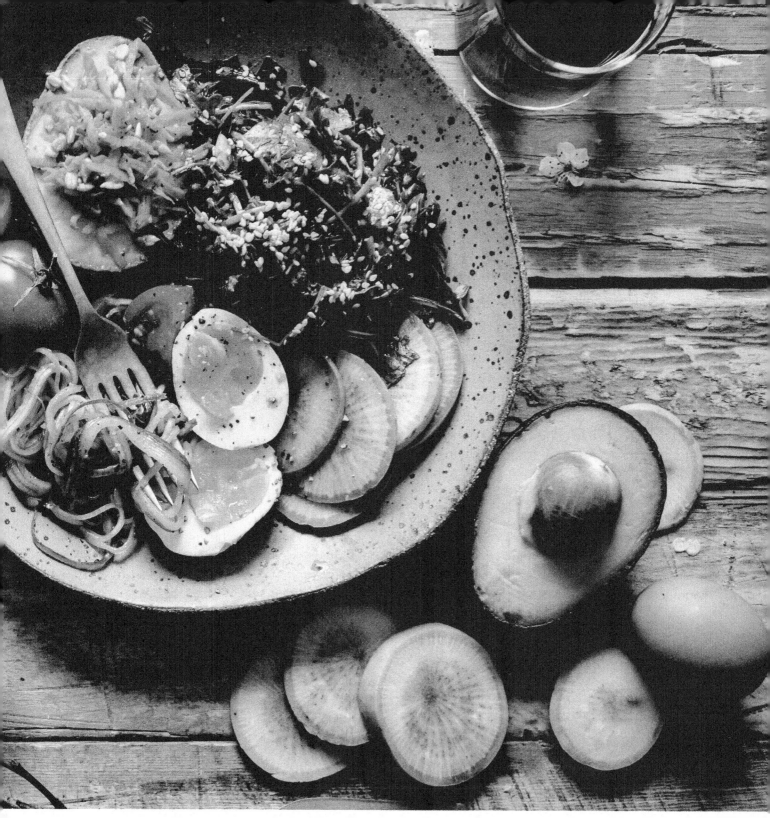

WHY EATING MORE FAT MAY LEAD TO MORE FAT BEING BURNED

There is ample evidence to suggest that fat loss occurs in people who adopt a ketogenic diet, however there has been much debate as to the exact mechanisms behind these effects. One theory is that consumption of carbohydrates results in a rise of insulin in the bloodstream. Insulin is the hormone responsible for the uptake of glucose and fatty acids into tissue cells, including adipose cells that store fat. Insulin also suppresses the breakdown of fat (lipolysis). Therefore, when blood insulin levels are low, there is an overall increase in the buildup of fat stores. This theory has been challenged, however, by findings that insulin is not solely responsible for fat uptake. Acylation stimulating protein (ASP) is actually released in response to fat intake in the diet and potently increases fatty acid uptake into adipose cells. There is also some debate as to whether insulin's effects are direct or whether uptake results from increased insulin release in response to ASP fat. This could possibly explain why not everyone who undergoes a ketogenic diet loses weight.

Another theory is based on the fact that, following a rapid increase in insulin levels, there is a drop, which induces a hunger response. When these insulin spikes and drops are not occurring, appetite is more tightly regulated. Additionally, people on a ketogenic diet may experience higher levels of satiety from protein intake and the appetite suppressant action of ketone bodies themselves. Ultimately, this leads to lower calorie intake and eventual fat loss.

The hypothesis that weight loss occurs because protein and fat digestion are more "expensive," or use more energy, than that of carbohydrates is also a popular theory. In the initial phases of the ketogenic diet, 16% of the glucose the body needs is produced by the body itself, through "gluconeogenesis," an energy-demanding process that converts glycerol and glycogenic amino acids from fat and protein into glucose. The energy required for this process comes from the breakdown of fat stores in the absence of glucose.

What is Vegetarianism?

A vegetarian can be defined as "a person who does not eat meat or fish, and also avoids other animal products, especially for moral, religious, or health reasons." It is more than a dietary choice; it is a lifestyle choice, which is often made after a lot of thought and with strong motives.

Much like the vegan diet, the vegetarian diet is plant-based, but unlike the vegan diet, only flesh from animals and fish are excluded. Within the broader category of vegetarianism are the ovo-vegetarians (those who do not eat meat but choose to eat eggs) and lacto-vegetarians (vegetarians who choose to eat dairy but not eggs and meat). Some vegetarians choose to eat both eggs and dairy. Other variations of plant-based diets include the pescatarian diet, which excludes all meat except fish and seafood. Some people also consider themselves "flexitarians" and follow a plant-based diet with occasional exceptions.

Becoming vegetarian is a personal choice. One reason an individual may choose the vegetarian lifestyle is morality. Many believe it is unethical to produce meat or fish products because animals suffer in the process. Increasingly, people are choosing to follow plant-based diets out of concern for the environment, since raising livestock contributes to the release of greenhouse gases. It also requires vast amounts of farmland and energy and can harm quality of life in many farmland communities around the world. Some religions such as Jainism, Hinduism, and Buddhism either require or advocate vegetarianism as a moral obligation.

It is important to carefully monitor nutrient consumption on a vegetarian diet because some nutrients that are readily available in meat and fish products are found in lower quantities in plants. One of the biggest concerns is adequate intake of protein. In the body, protein is broken down into its constituents, amino acids. Amino acids serve many vital functions; they are the structural components of many tissues and enzymes, which take part in biochemical processes critical to life.

Macronutrients

Macronutrients are nutrients that our bodies require in large amounts to provide energy. The three macronutrients are proteins, carbohydrates, and fats. Each macronutrient provides a different amount of energy per gram.

- 1 g protein = 4 calories
- 1 g carb = 4 calories
- 1 g fat = 9 calories

PROTEIN

The human body's structural components, including hair, nails, muscles, and organs, are all made up of protein. Protein from the diet is broken down into amino acids, which are then re-assimilated into protein structures. These structures are regularly undergoing repair. One example of such a protein structure is muscle, which is broken down during a workout, and repaired during the recovery period.

In addition to these structures, enzymes – proteins responsible for making chemical reactions in the body efficient – and antibodies – proteins responsible for the prevention of infection and disease – are also dependent on protein derived from the diet.

So it is clear that protein is vital for the body to function normally. If not enough protein is present in the diet, the body enters "starvation" mode and begins breaking down muscle fiber. It is therefore vital to consume sufficient protein.

It is important to note that while on a ketogenic diet, protein can act as an alternative source of glucose. Because it is the most efficient energy source, in the absence of carbohydrates, the body will seek to convert any extra protein available into glucose through a process called gluconeogenesis. So although this scenario is unlikely, since protein is less abundant in most plant sources than in meat, consuming too much protein can prevent ketosis even while following the ketogenic diet.

AMINO ACIDS

Amino acids are the building blocks of life. Individual amino acids serve critical functions. For example, tryptophan plays a role in the synthesis of serotonin, which regulates your mood, while arginine is used in the synthesis of nitric oxide to facilitate cardiovascular health.

Amino acids establish peptide bonds between them to form peptides and then polypeptides, which combine to make the protein structures that are a part of all the crucial chemical reactions that take place in your body, contributing to reproduction, metabolism, immunity, cell signaling, cell growth and differentiation, gene expression, anti-oxidative defense, and protein synthesis.

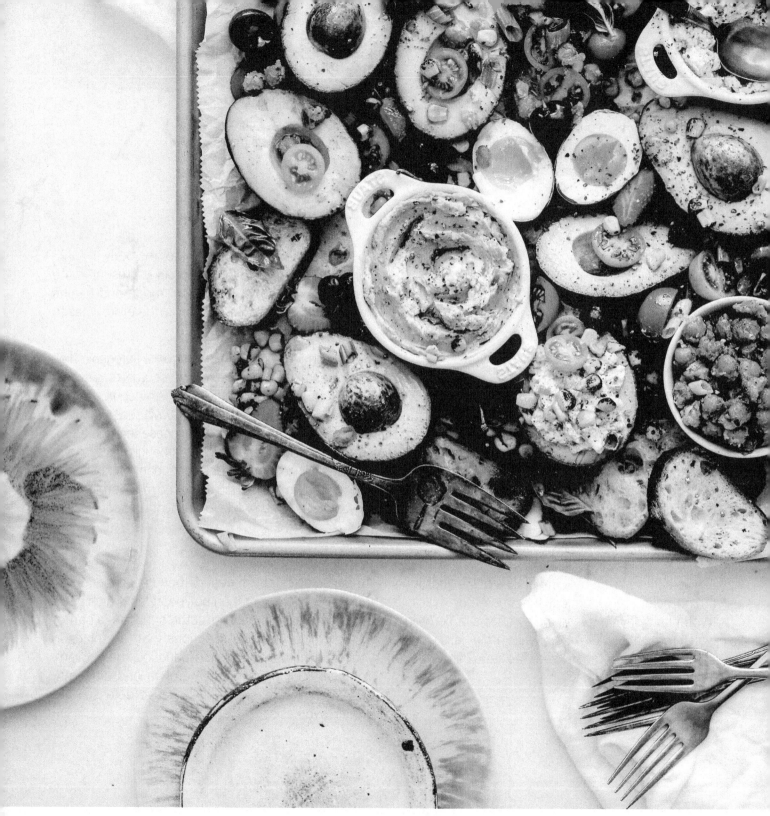

Twenty different kinds of amino acids are used to create proteins. Nine of the amino acids are known as "essential amino acids". These amino acids (methionine, leucine, isoleucine, histidine, lysine, phenylalanine, tryptophan, valine, and threonine) cannot be synthesized in the body and must be obtained from nutrition. The other amino acids (alanine, arginine, asparagine, aspartate/aspartic acid, cysteine, glutamine, glutamate/glutamic acid, glycine, proline, serine, and tyrosine) are classified as non-essential.

As non-essential amino acids are produced by the body from essential amino acids, it is important to ensure the required intake for all essential amino acids. If you don't consume the required levels of protein from which the essential amino acids are derived, a condition called hyperproteinemia (tissue degradation) can occur. As protein is more concentrated in meat and fish, the most common protein sources in typical western diets, being vegetarian requires extra vigilance to ensure all amino acids are acquired through a combination of diverse protein sources. Part of your body's mass is made up of protein, and amino acids carry out key bodily functions. An individual weighing 70kg generally has a protein make-up of around 12kg. These two numbers are used to calculate individual nutritional requirements to maintain body weight and monitor your plasma protein levels.

Vegetarian sources of protein include milk products (dairy), eggs, and of course, plant proteins. All protein found in animal products is originally derived from the nitrogen in plants that the animals consume, and although those plant proteins are less bioavailable to humans than animal proteins, which are structurally similar to our own, they still comprise a great source of protein. Soya is one such protein source that provides all essential amino acids. Exact recommended protein intake varies from country to country, however the estimated protein needs, according to the *American Journal of Clinical Nutrition*, are considered to be roughly 0.6g per kilogram of body weight.

THE IMPORTANCE OF LYSINE AND WHY YOU NEED TO GET ENOUGH OF IT

Lysine is one of the nine essential amino acids previously mentioned. It plays a crucial role as a building block of proteins. Lysine is needed for growth, as well as energy conversion and cholesterol level maintenance. This amino acid is converted in the human body to acetyl-CoA, which is a key factor in carbohydrate metabolism and energy production. It is also a precursor of carnitine, another amino acid responsible for the transportation of fatty acids that are used for energy production. Carnitine also has the ability to induce strong inflammatory and immune responses and plays a role in healing wounds and in inducing extensive angiogenic responses. Symptoms of a carnitine deficiency include:

- Fatigue
- Nausea
- Dizziness
- Anorexia
- Slow growth
- Anemia

How much Lysine do you need and how can you get it?

According to a joint report from the *World Health Organization*, the *Food and Agriculture Organization*, and *United Nations University,* 30mg per 1 kg of body weight of lysine should be consumed on a daily basis. This means approximately 2.1g for an individual weighing 70 kg. Vegetarians can get lysine from foods such as nuts, dairy products, and soy products like tofu. Lysine deficiency is rare, and it is important to note that a sharp rise in lysine amino acids in the body can lead to an increase in cholesterol and upset the stomach.

Lysine-rich vegetarian protein sources

Lysine is found in large amounts in meat and poultry, but there are also a wide variety of vegetarian options. Foods that contain high amounts of lysine include tempeh, tofu, soymilk black beans, pistachios, and of course, dairy products.

Tempeh	30g protein/cup	754mg lysine
Black beans	14g protein/cup	1046mg lysine
Soymilk	9g protein/cup	439mg lysine
Pistachios	12g protein/cup	734mg lysine
Seitan	6.7g protein/oz	219mg lysine
Skimmed Milk	8g protein/cup	40mg lysine
Parmesan Cheese	10.9g protein/oz	926mg lysine
Eggs	6g protein/egg	456mg lysine

CARBOHYDRATES

Carbohydrate molecules comprised of hydrogen, carbon, and oxygen are, as previously discussed, the body's preferred source of energy-efficient glucose.

Carbohydrates commonly found in the diet are sugar, fiber, and starch. Foods rich in carbohydrates are cheap to purchase and activate the body's reward system upon ingestion, which is why they are so popular. Many of the most commonly available carbohydrates lack micronutrients and serve simply as an energy source.

That said, not all carbohydrates are created equal. There are two types of carbohydrates: simple and complex. Simple carbohydrates, also known as simple sugars, are easily broken down during digestion because they are only made up of one or two units of sugar linked by glycosidic bonds. They include monosaccharides (glucose, fructose, and galactose) and disaccharides (lactose, sucrose, and maltose). They fall into the category of high-glycemic index foods that cause a rapid rise in blood sugar levels and subsequent insulin release. Examples of high-glycemic index foods are sodas, juices, and highly processed (refined) carbohydrates such as white bread, pasta, rice, breakfast cereals, crackers, pretzels, sweets, and desserts.

Complex carbohydrates are typically low- or medium-glycemic index foods and facilitate a much more gradual release of sugar into the bloodstream following a meal. This is because it takes longer to digest the oligosaccharide and polysaccharide chains that make up complex carbs. Examples of complex carbohydrate foods are whole wheat bread, oats, sweet potatoes/yams, corn, beans, peas and legumes, most fruits, as well as non-starchy vegetables like carrots. Complex carbs do not cause rapid insulin spikes and keep you satiated longer since they sit in the gut for longer periods of time during the digestion process. This leads to less frequent food intake, which ultimately results in less energy being stored as fat.

You should seek to consume more complex carbs than simple carbs. If you are following a gluten-free regimen, sources such as lentils, beans, and green peas are best.

FATS

Although fat has gotten a bad rep in the media over the past few decades, fat is actually a crucial component of our diet. Fat plays a vital role in the functioning of cells. We also need fat to absorb the fat-soluble vitamins A, D, E, and K. Fat serves as an insulator and offers protective functions to the internal organs.

Dietary fat is typically divided into two broader categories: saturated and unsaturated fats, with the latter being the healthier option due to their structures. They contain at least one double bond between their carbon molecules (monounsaturated) but often contain more (polyunsaturated). This introduces kinks in their carbon and hydrogen structures and gives them certain properties, like being liquid at room temperature, while saturated fats are solid. Consuming too much saturated fat can cause high cholesterol

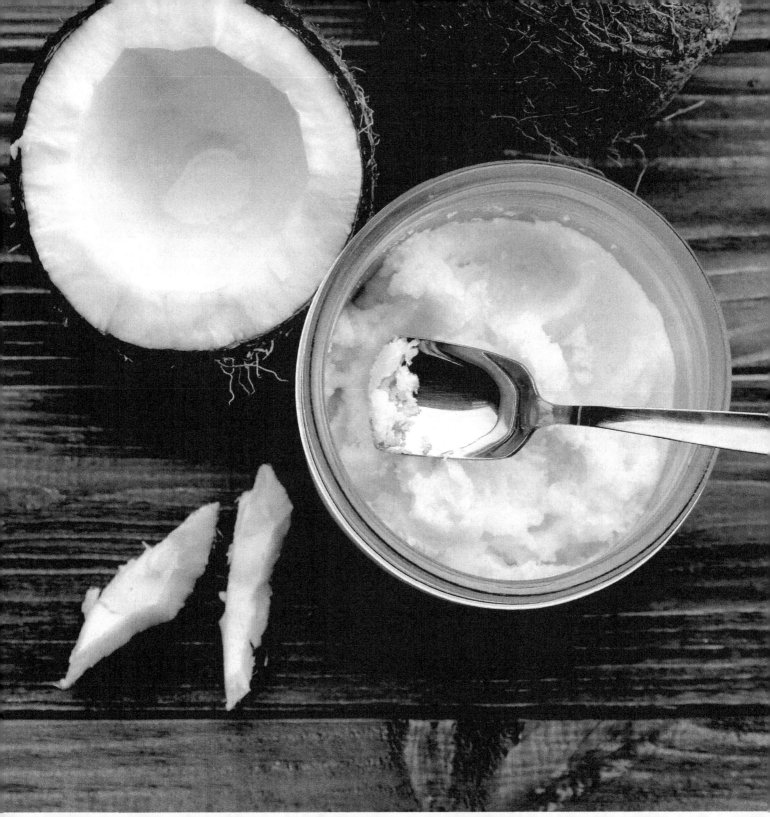

levels, which lead to health complications such as cardiovascular disease. Vegetarian sources of saturated fat are typically dairy products, though small amounts of saturated fats are also present in nuts and seeds. Eggs contain a balanced amount of both saturated and unsaturated fat. Unsaturated fats are found in avocados, nuts, seeds, and vegetable oils.

Olive oil, which offers several health benefits and can withstand high temperatures when heated, is a great, affordable source of fat. In comparison with butter and coconut oil, olive oil contains higher levels of monounsaturated fats than saturated fats and is the better option for those on a vegetarian diet. Other vegetable oils such as palm oil offer a more neutral contribution to the blood lipid profile. Despite containing high amounts of saturated fats, some of these oils, such as palmitic acid, have similar effects on the lipid profile as monounsaturated fats and contain cholesterol-lowering compounds.

A third category of fat that should be avoided at all costs is trans-fat. This is an unsaturated type of fat that is chemically hydrogenated into saturated fats to give them certain properties such as spreadability and an extended shelf life. The consumption of trans-fat increases the amount of harmful LDL cholesterol in the blood. It also reduces the beneficial HDL-levels. Avoid trans-fat even in the smallest amounts, as only 2% of daily calories derived from these fats can increase the risk to heart diseases by 23%.

Coconut Oil

As mentioned above, egg- and plant-based fats are key components for meeting fat needs in a vegetarian diet. One of these sources is coconut oil, which has been promoted for consumption and other uses in recent years. While coconut oil offers a very distinct and full flavor, the nutritional properties have been exaggerated. The available evidence that coconut oil lowers cardiovascular risk factors is weak, and there has been no clear indication that it improves lipid profiles. Reviews of the available literature suggest that unsaturated fats are a much better option when attempting to lower cardiovascular disease risk. Substitutes such as olive oil, hemp seed oil, and flax seed oil are better options to improve your lipid profile.

Healthy Oils and Fats

Perhaps the most significance reason to get the right balance of unsaturated and saturated fat in your diet is to optimize your blood lipid profile. A poor profile is a key risk factor in the development of metabolic syndrome, which is a cluster of biochemical and physiological abnormalities associated with the development of cardiovascular disease and type 2 diabetes. The consumption of monounsaturated and polyunsaturated fats contribute to the elevation of high-density lipoproteins (HDL) in the blood. This is often referred to as "good" cholesterol.

There has been a lot of controversy around the optimal intake levels of different fats. More recent studies have suggested that merely reducing the intake of "bad" cholesterol, or low-density lipoproteins, does not reduce an individual's coronary risk factor if HDL levels remain low. Insufficient omega-3 intake in particular carries a high CVD burden.

Besides keeping blood lipid profiles in balance, omega-3 fatty acids play a role in aiding brain function and in preventing asthma, certain cancers, and arthritis. While omega-3 fatty acids are most commonly found in fatty fish such as salmon and sardines, it is perfectly doable to satisfy your body's needs with vegetarian foods like chia or hemp seeds, flaxseed oils, brussels sprouts, and various nuts.

Getting the right ratio of omega-6s to omega-3s is important. Unlike omega-9s, these two fats cannot be produced by the body and must be derived from the diet in a ratio. The ideal ratio of 1:1 prevents inflammation, which is caused by higher intake of pro-inflammatory omega-6s.

According to various studies, 95 % of Americans have dangerously unbalanced omega-6 to omega-3 ratios, at around 15:1. Even an imbalance as small as 10:1 shows adverse health effects. With more careful monitoring of your diet, you will be able to achieve a more appropriate intake ratio through consumption of whole foods. Omega-6s can be found in seeds, nuts, green veggies, and oils, such as olive oil. To recap, consciously consuming foods such as flaxseed oil, hemp seeds, chia seeds, walnuts, and algal oil that are higher in omega-3s, which are less abundant in typical western diets, will help you to remain in balance.

Omega-9 fatty acids are a non-essential fatty acid since the body can produce it. Their production is dependent on sufficient levels of omega-6s and omega-3s, though they can also be found in avocados, nuts, chia seeds, and olive oil.

Since fats are energy-dense, overconsumption of any fat will result in energy imbalance and weight gain. The amount of energy taken in should be equal to or less than the energy expended. Everything in moderation!

Micronutrients

KETO-FLU AND MINERAL DEFICIENCIES

In the initial phases of the keto diet journey, there is the possibility of experiencing "keto-flu" owed to the effects of the drop in carbohydrate intake. It is crucial at this stage to carefully monitor electrolyte intake. A lack of magnesium and potassium can cause lethargy and, in extreme cases, lead to heart dysfunction.

POTASSIUM

The consumption of 3500 to 4700mg potassium per day potassium is recommended. A potassium deficiency can lead to hypokalemia, cardiac arrhythmia, muscle cramps, weakness, and anorexia. An avocado, which is low-carb, provides roughly 1000 mg of potassium. Spinach, zucchini, cauliflower, and yogurt are also great keto-vegetarian potassium sources. Depending on food sources, supplementing potassium is recommended on a ketogenic vegetarian diet.

It should be noted that too much potassium could be toxic, potentially causing hyperkalemia.

MAGNESIUM

Adult males should be consuming around 320-420mg magnesium per day. For adult females, the recommended amount per day is 300-400mg. Magnesium contributes to protein synthesis, the metabolism of glucose, muscle contraction, bone structure, and bone strength. The consumption of less than 300mg per day for an extended period can cause magnesium deficiency, resulting in muscle weakness and cramps, as well as cardiac arrhythmia.

Good natural sources of this mineral are dairy products, nuts, and dark, leafy greens. Supplementing is good idea if you're struggling to achieve proper dietary intake, but be aware that a maximum of 350 mg/day of magnesium in supplement form is tolerable.

The consumption of magnesium in large amounts is possibly unsafe. Symptoms of toxicity are nausea, vomiting and diarrhea.

SODIUM

The recommended intake of sodium is roughly 1500mg per day for the body to regulate its water and acid-base balance and to guarantee nerve functioning and muscle contraction. Symptoms of a deficiency include hyponatremia, nausea, anorexia, seizures, and in the worst cases, a coma.

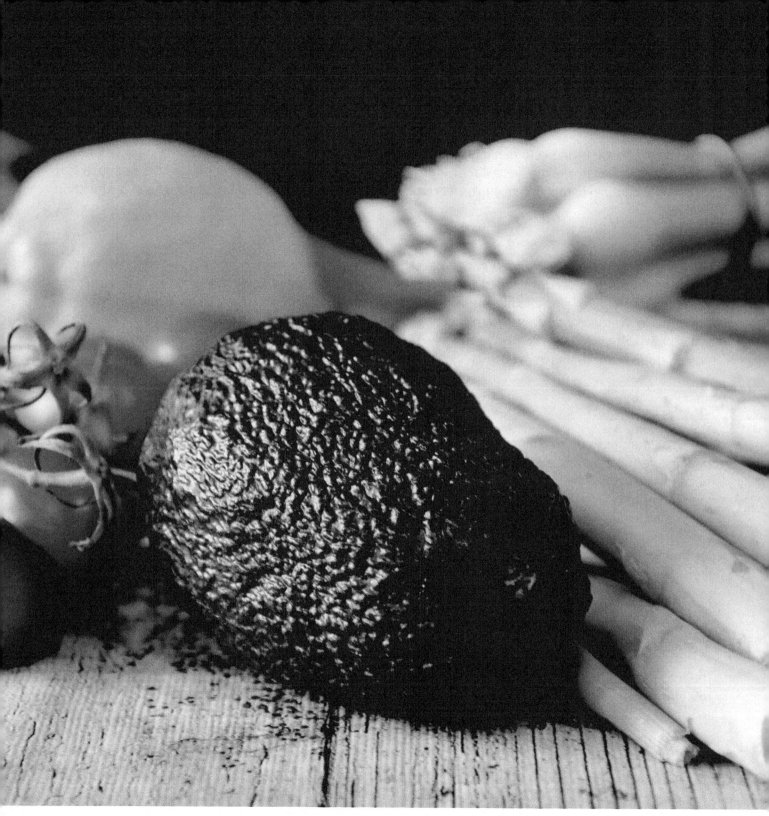

Some keto-vegetarian sodium sources include pickles, soy sauce, cheese, and actual salt, like Maldon, Himalayan, or table salt. It is just as important to get enough sodium as to avoid too much sodium, which can put your body at risk for kidney stones and some types of cancer.

CALCIUM

It is commonly known that calcium is important for the structure and strength of bones and teeth. Calcium also contributes to a healthy acid-base balance and takes part in nerve function, muscle contraction, blood clotting, and enzyme activation. Aim to consume roughly 1000mg per day. Great keto-vegetarian calcium sources include dairy products, leafy vegetables, soy milk, and almonds.

ZINC

Zinc plays an important role in protein synthesis, energy metabolism, immune functions, sensory functions, and the production of sex hormones. Women should aim to take in roughly 8mg per day, while males should aim for 11mg. Keto-vegetarian sources include eggs, dairy products, seeds, nuts, and nutritional yeast.

IRON

Iron is one of the most important dietary minerals because it plays a crucial role in oxygen delivery and is an essential component of the aerobic metabolism. Unfortunately, it is one of the more common deficiencies, particularly in women, vegetarians, and vegans. An iron deficiency is more common in vegetarians because iron from plant sources is less easily absorbed into the blood stream. It is important to ensure adequate vitamin C intake because this vitamin facilitates the absorption of iron in the gut. Common keto-vegetarian vitamin C sources include bell peppers, broccoli, strawberries, and dark, leafy greens.

The average iron needs for males is roughly 8mg per day while the requirement for females is closer to 18mg per day for proper functioning of the menstrual cycle. Good vegetarian sources include dark, leafy greens and small portions of dried fruit. Due to the poor absorption rates of iron from plant-based sources, consider iron supplements.

Note that polyphenols, phytates, and calcium can decrease the amount of iron absorbed. These elements are found in drinks life coffee and tea, and in grains, legumes, and dairy products. If you have an iron deficiency, it is best to avoid iron-containing ingredients that are also high in elements that compete with iron for absorption.

IODINE

Iodine is important for thyroid function. A deficiency is rarely a problem due to salt being fortified with Iodine. Most adults don't have trouble meeting the 150mg daily requirement, though in rare instances, severe deficiency can cause goiter.

PHOSPHORUS

Phosphorus requirements are roughly 700mg per day. This micronutrient promotes bone structure and strength, acid-base balance, and B-vitamin function. It is a component of the primary carrier of ATP, which stores and transports energy in cells. Sources include high-protein foods such as tofu and nuts. A deficiency is unlikely.

VITAMIN B12

The B12 vitamin is needed for important bodily functions such as protein metabolism and synthesis, fat and carbohydrate metabolism, neurotransmitter formation, and glycolysis. Vitamin B12 is more difficult to obtain on a vegetarian diet. Like complete amino acid profiles, it is more commonly found in meat and fish. Eggs, milk and cheese also contain B12, but in low quantities and it tends to be poorly absorbed.

Supplementation of B12 is a smart choice for vegetarians, and foods such almond milk are often fortified with vitamin B12. Consuming these products can help to ensure adequate intake, which is roughly 2.4-2.5mg per day.

A deficiency of vitamin B12 could lead to pernicious anemia, particularly in elderly people who have more trouble absorbing the vitamin. Being knowledgeable about vitamin B12 requirements and its functions will help you to make the right decisions for your health while following a ketogenic-vegetarian diet.

The Ketogenic Vegetarian Diet in Numbers

The ketogenic and vegetarian diets can be achieved in unison. A ketogenic vegetarian diet, simply put, is fat-rich and plant-based, but includes egg and dairy products. The consumption of carbohydrates should be minimized. A combination of both diets is slightly more challenging than the ordinary ketogenic diet, in which meat and fish can also be consumed for low-carb protein and fat.

To maintain a state of ketosis, the number of net carbs you can consume each day is limited to a recommended 30g. In order to achieve this, a strict meal plan is necessary. It is possible to consume up to 50g of carbohydrates and still lose weight, but this depends on calorie intake and goals of the individual. Since weight loss requires a calorie deficit, those aiming to lose bodyfat need to monitor calorie intake as well. The following is a breakdown of the percentages of macronutrients needed to formulate your diet more accurately:

- *5-10% of calories should come from carbs.*
- *15-30% of calories should come from protein.*
- *60-75% of calories should come from fatty foods.*

FIBER & NET CARBS

It is important to take a close look at the effects of fiber on blood glucose levels. There are two types of fiber: soluble fiber and insoluble fiber. The first can lower cholesterol levels and improve blood glucose, and the second keeps the digestive tract working well. You should aim to consume about 14 grams of fiber for every 1,000 calories to provide your body with these benefits. Foods like Chia seeds, berries, avocado, almonds, and various vegetables make it easy to obtain enough fiber from a keto-vegetarian diet.

Most people think that fiber does not affect blood sugar levels and that it doesn't contain calories. That's why many people only count the "net carbs" in a ketogenic dish: total carbs minus the fiber content. However, the US Food and Drug Administration (FDA) estimates that each gram of soluble fiber fermented by bacteria provides about 2 calories. Insoluble fibers are not digested at all, so the FDA estimates that they do not contribute any calories.

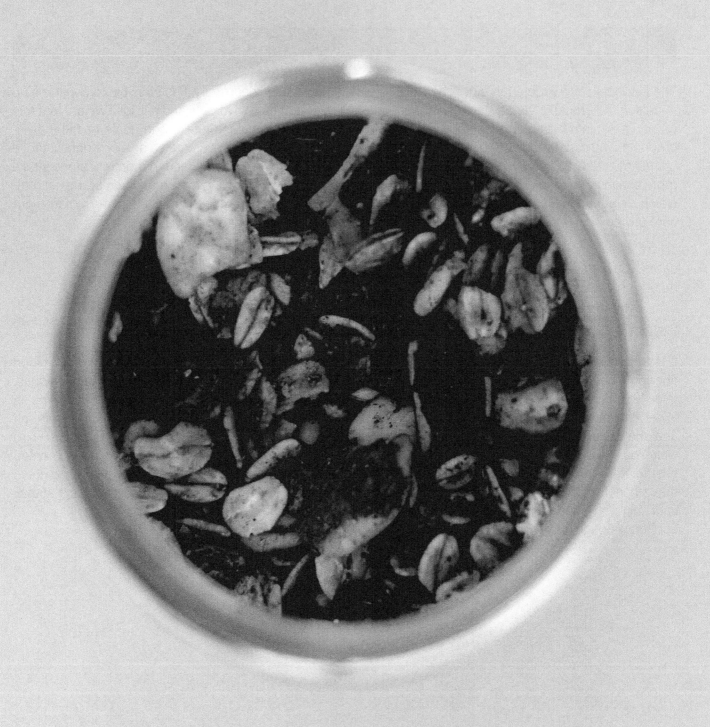

Low-Carb Vegetarian Foods

CARBS IN NUTS & SEEDS

If you make the decision to follow a ketogenic-vegetarian diet, it is useful to know the nutritional values of different nuts and seeds, as they tend to have fewer carbohydrates than other plant-based foods. They make a nice, portable snack, but be selective in choosing which to include in your diet, as a few are high in carbs (chestnuts, pistachios, and cashews).

The serving size has been set to 1 ounce to make it easy to calculate a larger serving.

Food	Serving	Metric	Fats(g)	Carbs(g)	Fiber(g)	Protein(g)	Net Carbs(g)
Chia seed	1 oz	28g	9	12	11	4	1
Pecan	1 oz	28g	20	4	3	3	1
Flax Seed	1 oz	28g	12	8	7	5	1
Brazil Nut	1 oz	28g	19	4	2	4	2
Hazelnut	1 oz	28g	17	5	3	4	2
Walnut	1 oz	28g	18	4	2	4	2
Coconut, Unsweetened	1 oz	28g	18	7	5	2	2
Macadamia Nut	1 oz	28g	21	4	2	2	2
Almond	1 oz	28g	15	5	3	6	2
Almond Flour	1 oz	28g	14	6	3	6	3
Pumpkin Seed	1 oz	28g	6	4	1	10	3
Sesame Seed	1 oz	28g	14	7	3	5	4
Sunflower Seed	1 oz	28g	14	7	3	6	4

CARBS IN GREENS

Vegetables are more or less the staple food of a healthy plant-based or vegetarian diet. Not all vegetables are low in carbohydrates, so it is important make sure to choose the right ones. Avoid those high in sugar and starch, and take extra caution with some greens, which can add a surprising amount of carbs to your diet if you do not monitor your intake.

Food	Serving	Metric	Fats(g)	Carbs(g)	Fiber(g)	Protein(g)	Net Carbs(g)
Endive	2 oz.	56g	0	2	2	1	0
Butter head Lettuce	2 oz	56g	0	1	0.5	1	0.5
Chicory	2 oz	56g	0	2.5	2	1	0.5
Beet Greens	2 oz	56g	0	2.5	2	1	0.5
Bok Choy	2 oz	56g	0	1	0.5	1	0.5
Alfalfa Sprouts	2 oz	56g	0	2	1	2	1
Spinach	2 oz	56g	0	2	1	1.5	1
Swiss Chard	2 oz	56g	0	2	1	1	1
Arugula	2 oz	56g	0	2	1	1.5	1
Celery	2 oz	56g	0	2	1	0.5	1
Chives	2 oz	56g	0	2.5	1.5	2	1
Collard Greens	2 oz	56g	0	3	2	1.5	1
Romaine lettuce	2 oz	56g	0	2	1	1	1
Asparagus	2 oz	56g	0	2	1	1	1
Eggplant	2 oz	56g	0	3	2	0.5	1
Radishes	2 oz	56g	0	2	1	0.5	1
Tomatoes	2 oz	56g	0	2	1	0.5	1

Food	Serving	Metric	Fats(g)	Carbs(g)	Fiber(g)	Protein(g)	Net Carbs(g)
White mushrooms	2 oz	56g	0	2	0.5	2	1.5
Cauliflower	2 oz	56g	0	3	1.5	1	1.5
Cucumber	2 oz	56g	0	2	0.5	0.5	1.5
Dill pickles	2 oz	56g	0	2	0.5	0.5	1.5
Bell green pepper	2 oz	56g	0	2.5	1	0.5	1.5
Cabbage	2 oz	56g	0	3	1	1	2
Fennel	2 oz	56g	0	4	2	1	2
Broccoli	2 oz	56g	0	3.5	1.5	1.5	2
Green Beans	2 oz	56g	0	4	2	1	2
Bamboo Shoots	2 oz	56g	0	3	1	1.5	2

CARBOHYDRATES IN FRUITS

The fruit of a plant is the reproductive organ that contains seeds. They are a popular food choice due their sweet taste. Okra, avocado, tomatoes, and green beans are in fact fruits, though many might think of them as vegetables. Avocados are an invaluable part of any keto diet as they are high in fat and low in carbohydrates.

Food	Serving	Metric	Fats(g)	Carbs(g)	Fiber(g)	Protein(g)	Net Carbs(g)
Rhubarb	2 oz	56g	0	2.5	1	1	1.5
Lemon Juice	1 oz	28g	0	2	0	0	2
Lime Juice	1 oz	28g	0	2	0	0	2
Raspberries	2 oz	56g	0	7	4	1	3
Blackberries	2 oz	56g	0	6	3	1	3
Strawberries	2 oz	56g	0	4	1	0	3

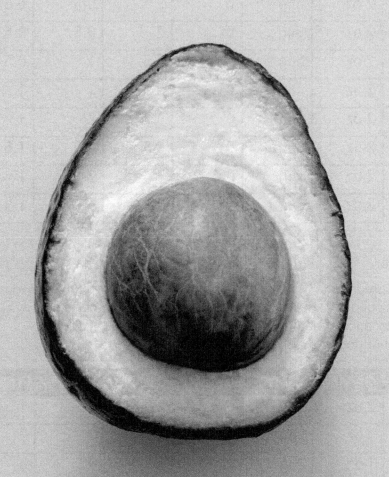

PROTEIN-RICH VEGETARIAN FOODS

Food	Serving	Metric	Fats(g)	Carbs(g)	Fiber(g)	Protein(g)	Net Carbs(g)
Tofu	3.5 oz	100g	5	2	1	16	1
Pumpkin seed	1 oz	28g	6	4	1	10	3
Almond	1 oz	28g	15	5	3	6	2
Flax Seed	1 oz	28g	12	8	7	5	1
Chia Seed	1 oz	28g	9	12	11	4	1
Brazil nut	1 oz	28g	19	4	2	4	2
Hazelnut	1 oz	28g	17	5	3	4	2
Walnut	1 oz	28g	18	4	2	4	2
Pecan	1 oz	28g	20	4	3	3	1
Unsweetened Coconut	1 oz	28g	18	7	5	2	2
Macadamia nut	1 oz	28g	21	4	2	2	2
Eggs	(1 egg)	50g	5	0	0	6	0
Milk (whole)	1 cup	250 ml	8	11	0	8	11
Cottage cheese	1oz	28g	1	1	0	4	1
Romano	1oz	28g	8	1	0	9	1
Non-fat cheddar	1oz	28g	2	0.5	0	7	0.5

FAT-RICH VEGETARIAN FOODS

As previously explored, monounsaturated and poly-unsaturated fats guarantee good cholesterol in the blood stream and should make up the majority of fats you consume. Remember that some saturated fat is needed, but in smaller amounts than unsaturated fat. Avoid trans-fat completely.

Food	Serving	Metric	Fats(g)	Carbs(g)	Fiber(g)	Protein(g)	Net Carbs(g)
Avocado oil	1 oz	28g	28	0	0	0	0
Cocoa butter	1 oz	28g	28	0	0	0	0
Coconut oil	1 oz	28g	28	0	0	0	0
Flaxseed oil	1 oz	28g	28	0	0	0	0
Macadamia oil	1 oz	28g	28	0	0	0	0
MCT oil	1 oz	28g	28	0	0	0	0
Olive oil	1 oz	28g	28	0	0	0	0
Red palm oil	1 oz	28g	28	0	0	0	0
Coconut cream	1 oz	28g	10	2	1	1	1
Olives, green	1 oz	28g	4	1	1	0	0
Avocado	1 oz	28g	4	2	2	1	0
Butter (ghee)	1oz	28g	23	0.2	0	0.2	0.2
Eggs	1 egg	50	5	0.4	0	6	0.4
Cheddar cheese	1 oz	28g	9	0.4	0	7	0.4
Red Leicester	1 oz	28g	9	0	0	6	0
Stilton	1 oz	28g	11	0	0	6	0

Losing Weight with a Ketogenic Vegan Diet

In order to lose weight, you must maintain a calorie deficit. This means that you must be burning more energy than you consume. A typical female will consume around 1700 calories daily when dieting, and for men this figure will be roughly 2200, though the ideal target of course differs according to each individual's height, weight, and activity level. To calculate how many daily calories you should be consuming, take the following steps:

1. Calculate your basal metabolic rate (BMR) using the following formula:
   - For men: BMR = (9.99 x weight in kilograms) + (6.25 x height in centimeters) - 4.92 x age in years + 5.
   - For women: BMR = (9.99 x weight in kilograms) + (6.25 x height in centimeters) - (4.92 x age in years) - 161.

2. Multiply your BMR by your activity factor:
   - If you engage in no exercise your activity factor is 1.2.
   - If you exercise one to three times a week, your activity factor is 1.375.
   - If you exercise three to five times per week, your activity factor is 1.55.
   - If you engage in heavy exercise six to seven times a week your activity factor is 1.72.
   - If you are an athlete or train heavily for sport and/or have a physically demanding job, your activity factor is 1.9.

The number you derive from this second calculation is the number of daily calories (kcal) you require to maintain your weight.

3. Take the figure you obtained from the calculation in step 2 and subtract 500kcal. The number you get will be the number of calories you should be consuming per week in order to lose roughly 0.5kg of fat in a week.

Consuming less than this would be irresponsible. The effects of consuming too few calories can wreak havoc on your body. When you suddenly start consuming much less than your body is used to, it can kick into "starvation mode" and start breaking down muscle instead of fat in an effort to ensure the body's needs are met. This muscle wasting will also show up as weight loss on the scale, but it goes without saying that this is not the goal you are attempting to achieve. You will retain your excess fat and lose muscle.

Below are some guidelines to help ensure you are not consuming too many calories for the keto-vegetarian diet:

- Be sure to combat cravings by taking advantage of the satiating effects of protein.
- Avoid making the mistake of snacking on too many nuts, seeds, and other fat-rich nibbles when trying to lose weight. These foods are very calorie-dense.
- If you have not seen any clear weight loss results after 2-3 weeks, you should consider monitoring your calorie intake closely.
- Be sure to enjoy the many non-starchy vegetables such as cauliflower, spinach, kale, broccoli, zucchini, and bell peppers, as well as fruits like avocados or berries. These contain many micronutrients in addition to being low in carbs.

How to test for ketosis

The body doesn't start burning fat as fuel the moment you lower your carb intake. That's why you want to start by aiming for nutritional ketosis. Once your body becomes fat-adapted, which happens after it has drained glycogen stores, it will start using fat as its main energy source. As a rule, especially at first, no more than five percent of your calories should come from carbohydrates. This means no more than 20g of net carbs on a 1600 kcal diet or 25g of net carbs on a 2000 kcal diet.

To guarantee ketosis, these strict numbers are not always required. After the first days or week of careful carb restriction, ketosis kicks in, and there will be some room for flexibility. Obviously, this doesn't mean reintroducing as many carbs as you want. To make sure your body maintains a state of ketosis, use the following testing methods.

Checking for acetate, acetoacetate, and beta-hydroxybutyrate can be done by testing your blood, breath, and urine. The preferred method is to test your urine using keto strips. Eventually, you'll find your optimal level where you feel best and notice progress.

To be absolutely sure, test your blood. By measuring millimoles per litre (mmol), you can accurately tell whether you're in ketosis or not. These values can be measured by a doctor or with a blood ketone meter.

- For nutritional ketosis mmol levels range from 0.5 to 1.0
- For optimal ketosis mmol levels range 1.5 to 3.0

Mental clarity, sustained energy, reduced cravings, and proper blood sugar levels are also positive signs of ketosis. Be careful when you're trying to add back more carbs to your diet; add only a very small number each week and check that your body is still running on fat as its main source of energy!

MACRONUTRIENT NUMBERS

The recipes you will find in this book include calorie and macro numbers. All calculations for these recipes have been done based on local ingredients. Ingredients around the world are generally the same, but different sources and manufacturing processes can result in slightly different nutrients present in your local ingredient. Do not worry about your local ingredients not meeting the ketogenic standards, but double checking from time to time doesn't hurt.

Epilepsy and Ketosis

Characterized by seizures, epilepsy is a neurological condition that can be difficult to diagnose because it has various causes that can be difficult to separate and identify. In addition, it can involve a range of case-dependent symptoms including:

- Seizures
- Stiffening of all muscles
- Loss of muscle control
- Repetitive jerking muscle movements
- Temporary loss of awareness
- Sensory disturbances and mood swings

Some typical causes of epilepsy are birth defects, brain tumors, brain injuries, or strokes. Roughly 1% of the world's population has epilepsy – around 65 million individuals – with 80% of the cases occurring in developing countries.

There are several treatment options available. Perhaps the most serious one is brain surgery, which is a very physically invasive and frightening process. This used to be a last resort but in more recently the procedure has become safer and more effective.

On the milder end of the treatment scale, diets have been applied to prevent seizures and have shown mixed results. One such diet is the ketogenic diet, which has been shown to be quite useful for the prevention of seizures, even though the mechanisms that cause the effects are unknown. Some research has explored the neuron-protecting effects of the ketogenic diet..

Alcohol on a Ketogenic Vegetarian Diet

Alcoholic drinks are often high in carbohydrates, so limiting your alcohol intake is advisable. Since alcohol is metabolized in the liver, where ketones are produced by the metabolism, it is possible for increased alcohol consumption to cause an increased output of ketone bodies. If you follow a ketogenic diet, you could therefore experience an increased "buzz" when consuming alcohol. Hangovers can also be intensified, and carb cravings may occur after alcohol intake. If you do have a drink, choose a hard liquor such as whiskey, rum, vodka, gin, or tequila. Avoid sugary alcoholic beverages like cocktails, and drink water along with the alcohol to mitigate its effects.

1. Flax Egg 🌿

Nutrition Information
(per serving)
- Calories: 37 kcal
- Net Carbs: 0.2 g.
- Fat: 2.7 g.
- Protein: 1.1 g.
- Fiber: 1.9 g.
- Sugar: 0 g.

INGREDIENTS:
- 1 tbsp. ground flaxseed
- 2-3 tbsp. lukewarm water

Total number of ingredients: 2

METHOD:
1. Mix the ground flaxseed and water in a small bowl by using a spoon.
2. Cover the mixture and let it sit for 10 minutes.
3. Use the flax egg immediately, or, store it in an air-tight container in the fridge and consume within 5 days.

Tip: You can use this mixture to replace a single egg in any recipe.

ESSENTIALS

2. Simple Marinara Sauce 🌿

Serves: 8 | Prep Time: ~20 min |

Nutrition Information
(per serving)
- Calories: 23 kcal
- Net Carbs: 2.8 g.
- Fat: 1.1 g.
- Protein: 0.7 g.
- Fiber: 0.9 g.
- Sugar: 0.1 g.

INGREDIENTS:

- 3 tbsp. olive oil
- 1 14-oz. can peeled tomatoes (no sugar added)
- ⅓ cup red onion (diced)
- 2 garlic cloves (minced)
- 2 tbsp. oregano (fresh and chopped, or 1 tbsp. dried)
- ½ tsp. cayenne pepper
- Salt and ground black pepper to taste
- Optional: 1 tbsp. sunflower seed butter (use grass-fed butter for a lacto sauce)

Total number of ingredients: 9

METHOD:

1. Heat the olive oil in a medium-sized skillet over medium heat.

2. Add the onions, garlic, salt, and cayenne pepper. Sauté the onions until translucent while stirring the ingredients.

3. Add the peeled tomatoes and more salt and pepper to taste.

4. Stir the ingredients, cover the skillet, and allow the sauce to softly cook for 10 minutes.

5. Add the oregano, and if desired, stir in the optional butter.

6. Take the skillet off the heat. The sauce is now ready to be used in a recipe!

7. Alternatively, store the sauce in an airtight container in the fridge and consume within 3 days. Store for a maximum of 30 days in the freezer and thaw at room temperature.

Tip: Use fresh herbs. Add a handful of chopped basil, parsley, or thyme for more flavor!

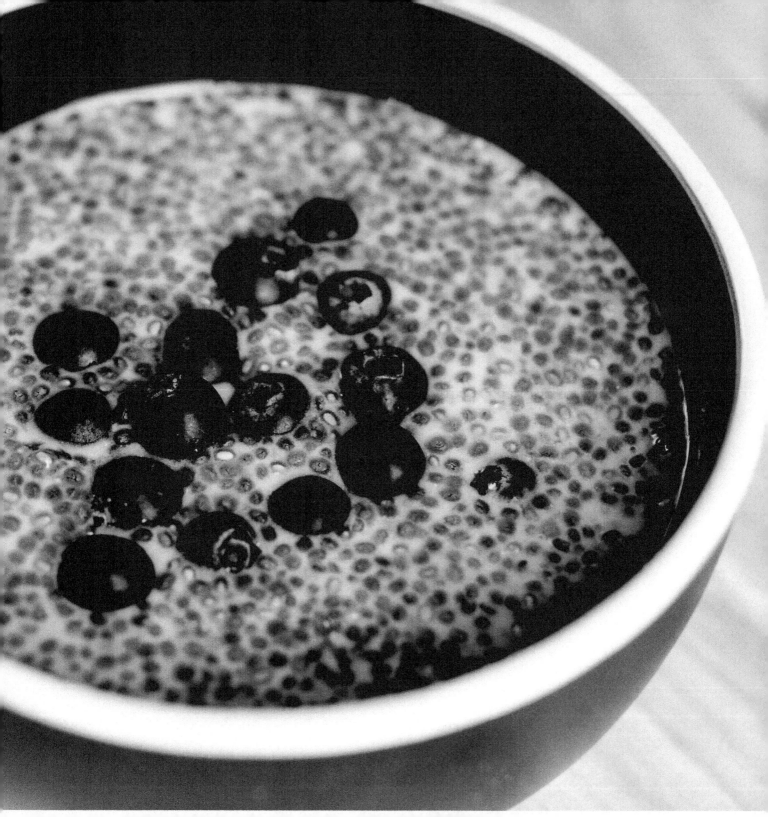

1. Chia Pudding with Blueberries 🍃

Serves: 2 | Prep Time: ~15 min |

Nutrition Information
(per serving)
- Calories: 256 kcal
- Net Carbs: 6.2 g.
- Fat: 19.8. g
- Protein: 9.6 g.
- Fiber: 21.9 g.
- Sugar: 1.8 g.

INGREDIENTS:
- 12 tbsp. chia seeds
- 3 cups unsweetened almond milk
- 1 cup water
- 4-6 drops stevia sweetener
- ¼ cup blueberries

Total number of ingredients: 5

METHOD:

1. Put all the ingredients in a medium-sized bowl and stir. Alternatively, put all ingredients in a mason jar, close tightly, and shake.

2. Allow the pudding to sit for 5 minutes, then give it another stir (or shake).

3. Transfer the bowl or mason jar to the fridge. Refrigerate the pudding for at least 1 hour.

4. Give the pudding another stir, top it with the blueberries, and then serve and enjoy!

5. Alternatively, store the pudding in an airtight container in the fridge and consume within 4 days. Store for a maximum of 30 days in the freezer and thaw at room temperature.

Note: This chia seed pudding is a great breakfast dish and can be prepared the night before serving. Simply allow the pudding to refrigerate overnight.

Tip: Mix up the combination of berries. Any low-carb fruit, like raspberries or strawberries, can be used as an addition to or substitute for blueberries!

BREAKFASTS

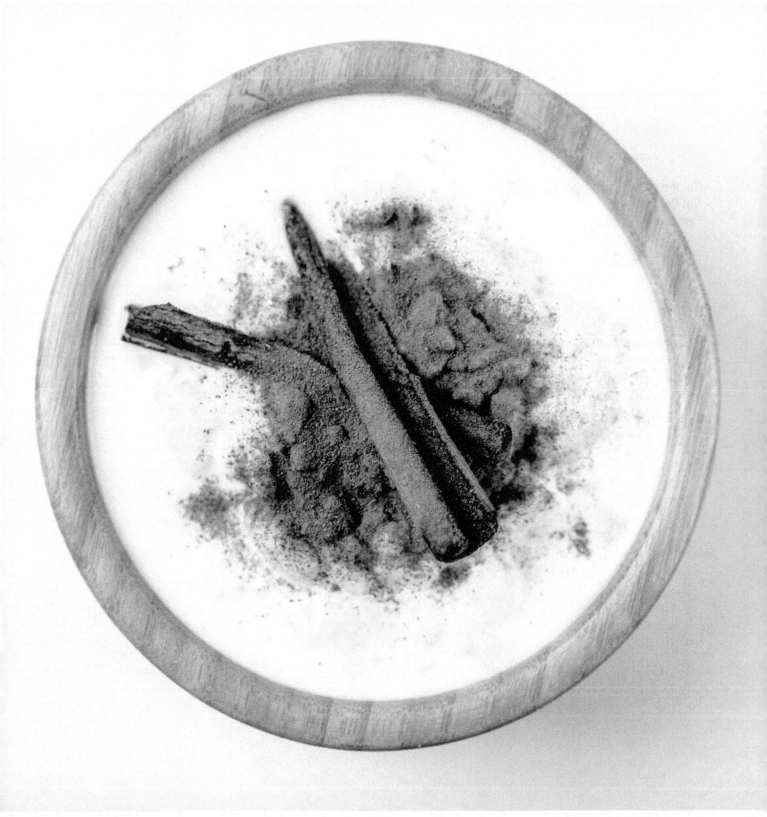

2. Coconut Porridge

Nutrition Information
(per serving)
- Calories: 357 kcal
- Net Carbs: 5.15 g.
- Fat: 32.9 g.
- Protein: 8.3 g.
- Fiber: 11.3 g.
- Sugar: 3 g.

INGREDIENTS:

- ¼ cup dried coconut (unsweetened)
- ½ cup full-fat coconut milk (unsweetened)
- ⅔ cup water (or more depending on consistency)
- 3 tbsp. coconut flour
- 2 tbsp. psyllium husk
- ¼ tsp. vanilla extract
- 3-6 drops stevia sweetener (or more depending on the desired sweetness)
- Pinch of cinnamon
- Pinch of nutmeg
- 4 tbsp. toasted almond flakes
- Optional: pinch of salt

Total number of ingredients: 11

METHOD:

1. Put a medium-sized pot over medium-high heat.
2. Toast the dried coconut in the pot while stirring for about 2 minutes.
3. Stir in the water and coconut milk.
4. Cover the pot and bring the mixture to a boil. Continue to stir in the remaining ingredients except the almond flakes.
5. Remove the pot from the heat and transfer the porridge to medium-sized bowls.
6. Top it with the almond flakes, some additional cinnamon, and enjoy!
7. Alternatively, store the porridge in an airtight container in the fridge and consume within 4 days. Store for a maximum of 60 days in the freezer and thaw at room temperature.

Note: Substitute the vanilla extract and sweetener with a scoop of vanilla flavored organic soy protein powder. This will add protein and make the dish even more ketogenic-proof!

Tip: This dish can also be prepared in an instant pot. Simply add the ingredients—except the almond flakes—and set the pot to cook the porridge right before waking up!

3. Eggless Handvo 🍶

Serves: 1 | Prep Time: ~20 min |

Nutrition Information
(per serving)
- Calories: 280 kcal
- Net Carbs: 6.8 g.
- Fat: 23.4 g.
- Protein: 9.3 g.
- Fiber: 7.9 g.
- Sugar: 2.3 g.

INGREDIENTS:

Mixture:
- ¼ cup chopped gourd (calabash, canned or fresh)
- ¼ cup paneer (ground)
- ½ tbsp. ginger (grated)
- 2 green chilis (diced)
- ½ tsp. salt
- 4-6 drops stevia sweetener
- ½ tsp. citric acid
- ½ tbsp. olive oil
- ¼ tsp. red chili powder
- ¼ tsp. turmeric powder
- ¼ tsp. asafoetida
- 2 tbsp. almond flour
- ½ tbsp. flaxseed flour or meal
- 1 tbsp. psyllium husk
- 1 tbsp. hung curd
- ¼ tsp. baking soda
- Optional: water

Preparation:
- ½ tbsp. olive oil
- 1 tbsp. mustard seeds
- 1 green chili (diced)
- 3 fresh curry leaves
- ½ tsp. sesame seeds
- 1 tsp. coriander leaves (chopped)

Total number of ingredients: 23

METHOD:

1. Put all the mixture ingredients—except the flours—in a food processor. Blend the ingredients into a smooth mixture. If necessary, add some water.
2. Transfer the mixture to a medium-sized bowl and incorporate the flours. Stir well until a batter is formed.
3. Take a medium-sized skillet, add ½ tablespoon of olive oil, and put it over medium heat.
4. Add the remaining preparation ingredients while stirring.
5. Then add the mixture ingredients, flatten out, and cover the skillet with a lid.
6. Cook the handvo for 5 minutes.
7. Carefully flip the handvo by flipping the skillet while covering it with a plate. Slide the flipped handvo on the plate back into the skillet.
8. Cover the skillet again and cook the handvo for another 5 minutes before serving and enjoy.
9. Alternatively, store the handvo in an airtight container in the fridge and consume within 3 days. Store for a maximum of 30 days in the freezer and thaw at room temperature.

Note: Handvo is a traditional Indian dish, and some of the ingredients might be difficult to find. Try Indian or Asian food stores.

Tip: Less water is better. Use a food processor for the best blending results.

4. Protein Nut 'N Seed Bread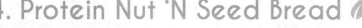

Nutrition Information
(per serving)
- Calories: 393 kcal
- Net Carbs: 4.3 g.
- Fat: 35.2 g.
- Protein: 13.8 g.
- Fiber: 6.6 g.
- Sugar: 1.7 g.

INGREDIENTS:
- ¼ cup almonds
- ¼ cup hazelnuts
- ½ cup pumpkin seeds
- ¼ cup flax seeds
- 3 flax eggs ()
- 3 tbsp. sesame seeds
- 3 cups almond flour
- 1 scoop organic soy protein powder (unflavored; or alternatively, use vanilla flavor)
- 2 tbsp. coconut flour
- 1½ tsp. baking soda
- Pinch of salt
- ½ cup unsweetened almond milk
- 1 tbsp. apple cider vinegar
- ⅓ cup coconut oil
- 2 tbsp. low-carb maple syrup
- 2 tbsp. water (or more depending on dough consistency)

Total number of ingredients: 16

METHOD:
1. Preheat the oven to 350°F / 180°C.
2. Line a loaf pan with parchment paper.
3. Put the almonds and hazelnuts in a blender or food processor. Pulse until ground.
4. Add the seeds and blend the ingredients again until ground. Scrape the sides of the blender or food processor if necessary.
5. Transfer the mixture to a large bowl and mix in the almond flour, baking soda, and salt with a whisk or spoon.
6. Take a separate medium-sized bowl and add the almond milk, protein powder, flax eggs, coconut oil, maple syrup, and vinegar. Stir well until all the ingredients are incorporated. Add 2 table-spoons of water (or more, if necessary), and stir.
7. Allow the wet mixture to sit for a few minutes. Stir again and then add it to the dry mixture in the large bowl.
8. Use a whisk or spoon to combine all ingredients.
9. Transfer the dough to the loaf pan lined with parchment paper.
10. Put the loaf pan in the oven and bake the bread for 50 minutes or until a fork comes out clean. Take the pan out of the oven and allow the bread to cool down.
11. Remove the parchment paper, transfer the bread to a cutting board, and slice it into 10 slices before serving. Enjoy!
12. Alternatively, store the bread in an airtight container in the fridge and consume within 5 days. Store for a maximum of 60 days in the freezer and thaw at room temperature.

Note: You can substitute almonds for hazelnuts and vice versa. You can also substitute hazelnut flour for the almond flour, or use a mixture of both.

Tip: Add more seeds and crushed nuts on top of the dough. Use a protein powder with little-to-no flavor. Serve this bread for Guacamole and Full-Fat Egg Salad (page 80) or Avocado and Cauliflower Hummus (page 79)!

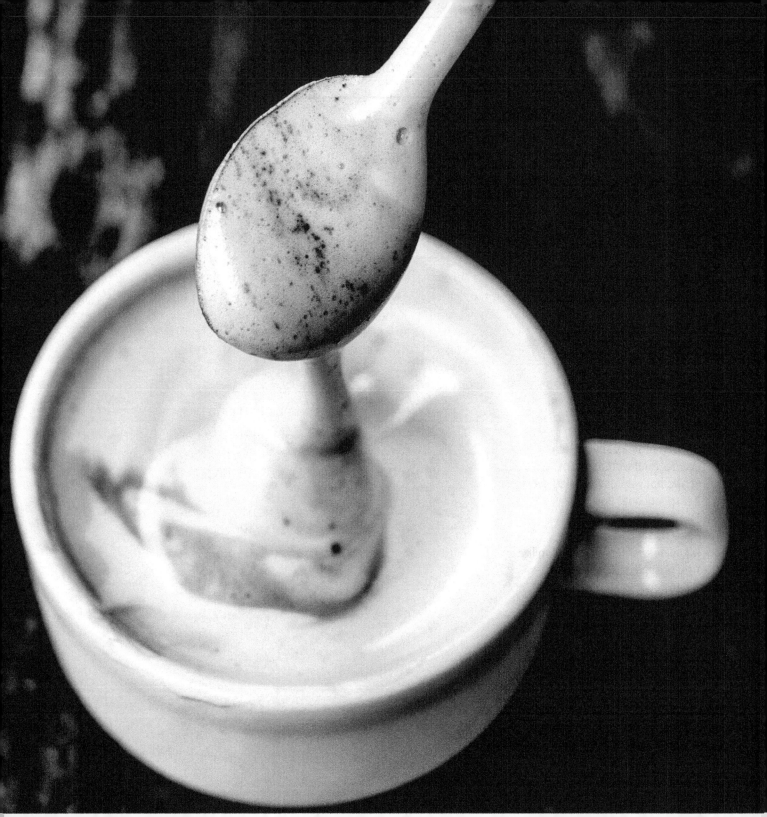

5. Special Egg Coffee

Serves: 4 | Prep Time: 20 min |

Nutrition Information
(per serving)
- Calories: 178 kcal
- Net Carbs: 1.9 g.
- Fat: 17.4 g.
- Protein: 3.5 g.
- Fiber: 0 g.
- Sugar: 0.5 g.

INGREDIENTS:

Low-Carb Condensed Milk:
- ½ cup heavy whipping cream
- 1 tbsp. grass-fed butter (unsalted)
- 12 drops stevia sweetener
- 1 tsp. pure vanilla extract
- Pinch of salt

Coffee:
- 4 cups of black coffee
  (use Vietnamese coffee if available)
- 4 egg yolks
- Optional: ½ tsp. pure vanilla extract

Total number of ingredients: 8

METHOD:

1. Add all the low-carb condensed milk ingredients—except the vanilla extract—to a small saucepan and put it over medium heat. Allow the mixture to simmer for up to 15 minutes while occasionally stirring with a spoon.

2. Remove the saucepan from the heat and stir in the teaspoon of vanilla extract.

3. Take a small bowl and whisk the egg yolks in it.

4. Add one tablespoon of the low-carb condensed milk to the yolks and stir. Continue this one tablespoon at a time until all condensed milk is mixed with the yolks.

5. Beat the mixture for a few minutes with a whisk until it starts to thicken.

6. Make sure to use hot coffee, and serve in large coffee cups.

7. Divide the egg mixture evenly between the 4 cups of coffee by carefully pouring on top of each. Serve the special egg coffee, topped with the optional vanilla extract if desired, and enjoy!

8. Alternatively, store the coffee in an airtight container or mason jar in the fridge and consume within 1 day.

Tip: To serve this coffee the traditional way, put the coffee cup in a medium-sized bowl filled with boiled water.

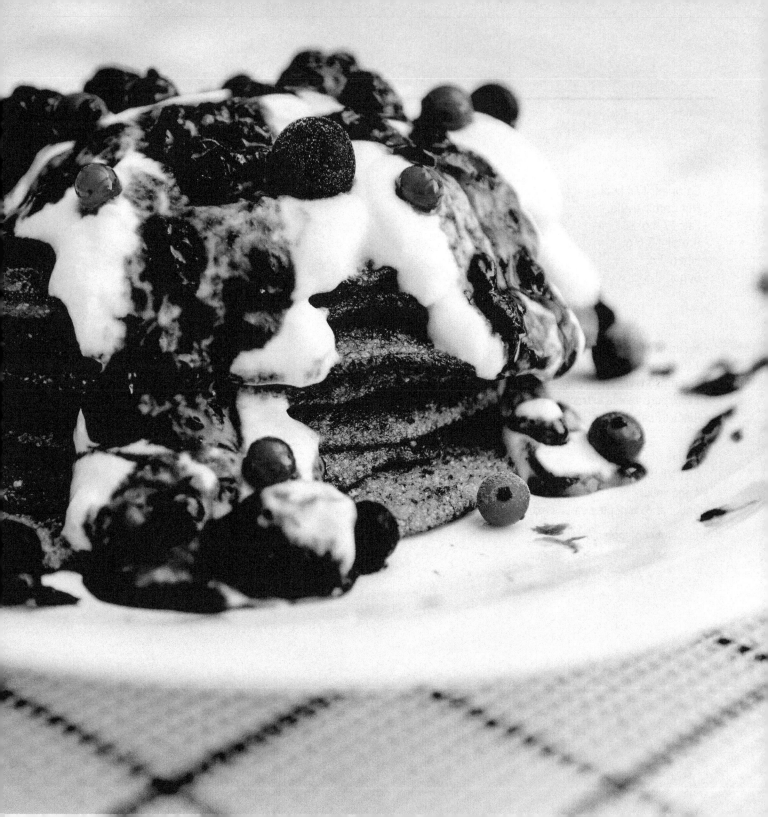

6. Yogurt & Berry Pancakes

Nutrition Information
(per serving)
- Calories: 452 kcal
- Net Carbs: 5 g.
- Fat: 41 g.
- Protein: 15.7 g.
- Fiber: 0.3 g.
- Sugar: 2.6 g.

INGREDIENTS:

Pancakes:

- 4 large organic eggs
- 1 cup cream cheese
- ¼ cup grass-fed butter
- 1 scoop organic soy protein powder
  (vanilla or chocolate flavor)
- 1 tsp. cocoa powder (unsweetened)
- Optional: ½ tsp. vanilla extract
- 4 tbsp. olive oil
  (or alternatively, use coconut oil)

Toppings:

- ¼ cup blueberries (or raspberries)
- 1 cup full-fat Greek yogurt

Total number of ingredients: 9

METHOD:

1. Take a medium-sized bowl and add the butter and eggs. Beat these ingredients for 2 minutes until incorporated by using a whisk.

2. Add the cream cheese, protein powder, cocoa powder, and if desired, the optional vanilla extract.

3. Mix all ingredients together for about 4 minutes, until no lumps remain.

4. Take a small skillet, put it over medium heat, and add 1 tablespoon of olive oil.

5. Transfer up to 4 tablespoons of the mixture to the pan and cook it for 2-3 minutes.

6. Flip the pancake and cook it for an additional 2 minutes.

7. Repeat steps 4, 5, and 6 until there is no mixture left.

8. Add 2 or more tablespoons of Greek yogurt to each pancake, garnish it with a few blueberries on top before serving, and enjoy!

9. Alternatively, store the pancakes and the toppings (separated) in the fridge, using an airtight container and consume within 3 days. Store for a maximum of 30 days in the freezer and thaw at room temperature. Use a microwave, toaster oven, or pan to reheat the pancakes.

Tip: Using a tablespoon of oil per pancake can help to reach your daily calories on a low-carb diet. Use less oil if desired.

7. Greek Chia Pudding 🍼

Serves: 3 | Prep Time: ~20 min |

Nutrition Information
(per serving)
- Calories: 318 kcal
- Net Carbs: 6.5 g.
- Fat: 26.6 g.
- Protein: 11.9 g.
- Fiber: 7.4 g.
- Sugar: 4 g.

INGREDIENTS:
- 1 cup full-fat Greek yogurt
- ½ cup full-fat coconut milk
- ½ scoop organic soy protein powder (vanilla or chocolate flavor)
- 5 tbsp. chia seeds
- 4-6 drops stevia sweetener (or alternatively, use low-carb maple syrup)
- ¼ cup raspberries
- ¼ cup pecans (crushed)
- Optional: 1-2 tbsp. water

Total number of ingredients: 8

METHOD:
1. In a medium-sized bowl, mix the yogurt with the coconut milk.
2. Stir in the protein powder and chia seeds until the protein powder is fully incorporated. Add some water if necessary.
3. Allow the pudding to sit for 2 minutes; then add the stevia sweetener and give the yogurt another stir.
4. Refrigerate the pudding overnight (or for at least 8 hours). This will guarantee a perfect pudding.
5. Top the pudding with the raspberries and crushed pecans; serve and enjoy!
6. Alternatively, store the pudding in an airtight container and keep it in the fridge and consume within 4 days. Or, you can freeze the pudding for a maximum of 30 days and thaw at room temperature.

Tip: You can add more coconut milk or water with chia seeds in proportion. Substitute the raspberries with blueberries or sliced strawberries!

8. Greek Yogurt Smoothie Bowl 🍶

Serves: 2 | Prep Time: ~75 min |

Nutrition Information
(per serving)
- Calories: 300 kcal
- Carbs: 18 g.
- Net Carbs: 8 g.
- Fat: 22.4 g.
- Protein: 15 g.
- Fiber: 10 g.
- Sugar: 4 g.

INGREDIENTS:

Smoothie:
- ¼ cup chia seeds
- 1 cup unsweetened almond milk
- ½ cup water
- ½ cup full-fat Greek yogurt
- ¼ cup mixed berries (frozen;
  or alternatively, use fresh berries)
- ½ scoop organic soy protein powder
  (vanilla flavor)
- 1-2 ice cubes
  (depending on desired consistency)

Toppings:
- ¼ cup almonds (crushed)
- 4-6 drops stevia sweetener
- ¼ cup toasted coconut flakes
- Optional: 2 tbsp. chia seeds

Total number of ingredients: 11

METHOD:

1. Mix the chia seeds with the almond milk and water in a medium-sized bowl.

2. Allow the mixture to sit for 2 minutes, then stir again; refrigerate, covered, for 1 hour.

3. Transfer the mixture to a blender and add the Greek yogurt, mixed berries, protein powder, and ice cubes.

4. Blend the ingredients on low speed until all ingredients are incorporated. Make sure that no lumps remain.

5. Transfer the smoothie to 2 serving bowls and garnish with the topping ingredients.

6. If desired, finish with the optional topping of 2 tablespoons of chia seeds. Refrigerate the smoothie bowl for an additional 10 minutes before serving and enjoy!

7. Alternatively, store the smoothie in an airtight container or mason jar, keep it in the fridge, and consume within 3 days. Store for about 30 days in the freezer and thaw at room temperature.

Tip: Add more toppings, like blueberries, crushed pecans, and/or almonds.

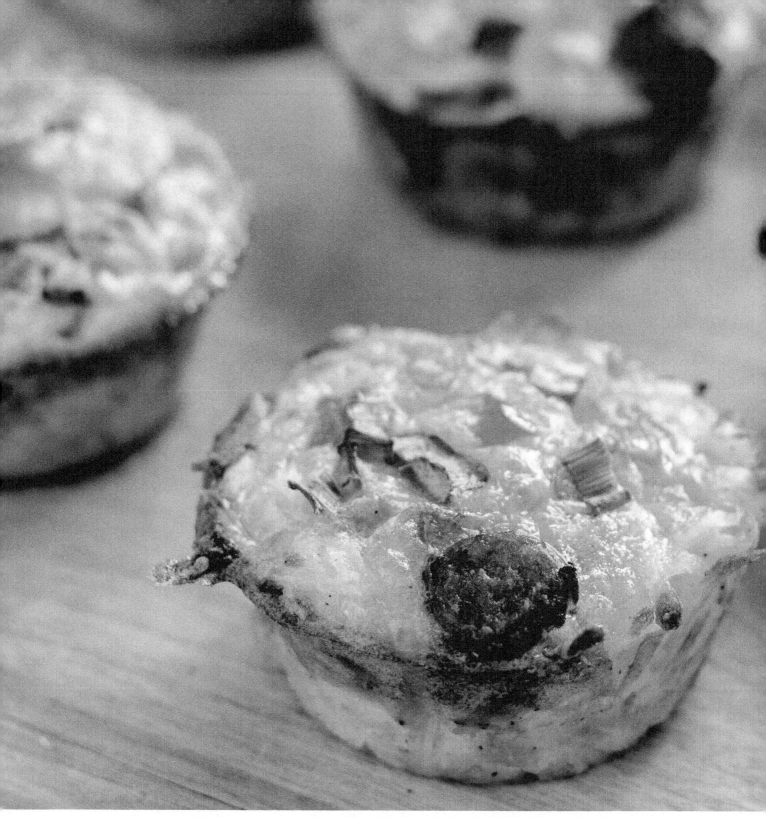

9. Eggfast Muffins 🥚

Serves: 9 | Prep Time: ~40 min |

Nutrition Information
(per serving)
- Calories: 76 kcal
- Net Carbs: 1.1 g.
- Fat: 4.9 g.
- Protein: 6.9 g.
- Fiber: 0.4 g.
- Sugar: 0.6 g.

INGREDIENTS:
- 9 large organic eggs
- 1 cup mushrooms (sliced)
- ½ cup scallions (finely chopped)
- 1 cup broccoli florets (stems removed)
- 4 tbsp. sugar-free sweet hot sauce
- Sea salt and pepper to taste
- ¼ cup fresh parsley (chopped)

Total number of ingredients: 8

METHOD:

1. Preheat oven to 375°F / 190°C, and line a 9-cup muffin tray with muffin liners.

2. Take a large bowl, crack the eggs in it, and whisk while adding salt and pepper to taste.

3. Add all the remaining ingredients to the bowl and stir thoroughly.

4. Fill each muffin liner with the egg mixture. Repeat this for all 9 muffins.

5. Transfer the tray to the oven and bake for about 30 minutes, or until the muffins have risen and browned on top.

6. Take the tray out of the oven, and let the muffins cool down for about 2 minutes; serve and enjoy.

7. Alternatively, store the muffins in an airtight container in the fridge, and consume within 3 days. Store for a maximum of 30 days in the freezer and thaw at room temperature. Use a microwave, toaster oven, or pan to reheat the omelet.

Tip: add ¼ cup of chopped jalapenos to the egg mixture and top each muffin with halved cherry tomatoes for a delicious variation!

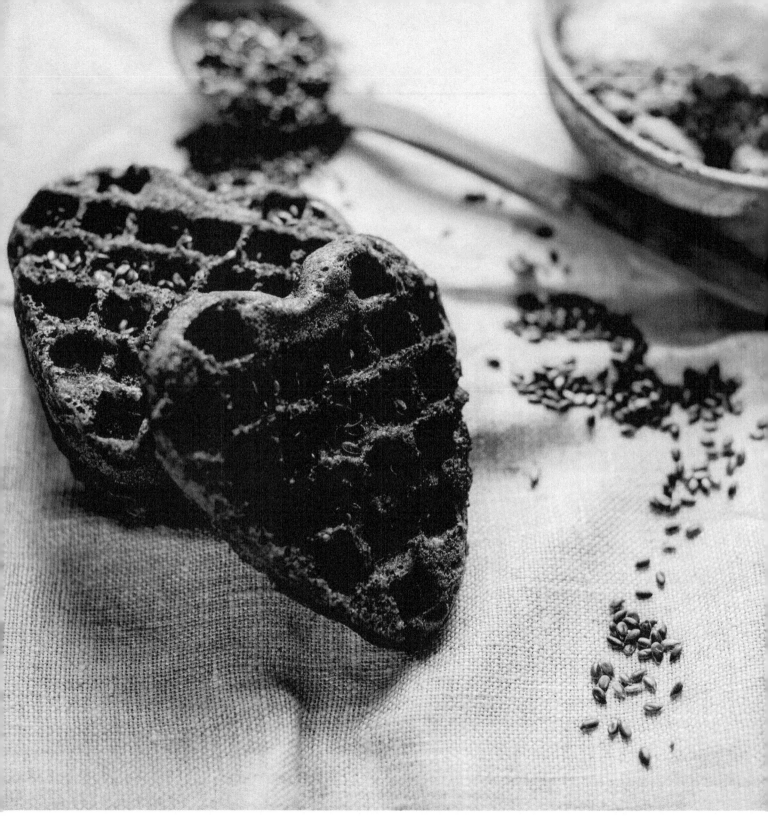

10. Crispy Flaxseed Waffles

Serves: 8 | Prep Time: 35 min |

Nutrition Information
(per serving)
- Calories: 204 kcal
- Net Carbs: 1.5 g.
- Fat: 18 g.
- Protein: 8 g.
- Fiber: 5.9 g.
- Sugar: 0.3 g.

INGREDIENTS:
- 2 cups golden flaxseed
  (if available, use golden flaxseed meal)
- 1 tbsp. baking powder
- 5 large organic eggs (for vegan waffles,
  replace with 5 flax eggs)
- ½ cup water (slightly more if necessary)
- ⅓ cup extra virgin olive oil
- 1 tbsp. ground cinnamon
- 1 tbsp. pure vanilla extract
- 6-12 drops stevia sweetener
  (or more depending on desired sweetness)
- Pinch of salt
- Optional: ¼ cup toasted coconut flakes

Total number of ingredients: 10

METHOD:
1. Preheat a waffle maker. If you don't have a waffle maker, heat a medium-sized skillet over medium-high heat for crispy flaxseed pancakes. Grease the waffle maker or skillet with a pinch of olive oil.

2. Take a medium-sized bowl and combine the flaxseed (or flaxseed meal) with the baking powder, eggs, water, remaining olive oil, and a pinch of salt. Incorporate all ingredients by using a whisk and allow the mixture to sit for 5 minutes.

3. Transfer the mixture to a blender or food processor and blend until foamy.

4. Pour the mixture back into the bowl and allow it to sit for another 3 minutes.

5. Add the remaining dry ingredients—except the optional toasted coconut flakes—and incorporate everything by using a whisk.

6. Scoop ¼ of the mixture into the waffle maker or skillet. Cook until a firm waffle or pancake has formed. When using a skillet, carefully flip the pancake.

7. Repeat this process for the 3 remaining parts of the batter.

8. Serve the waffles (or pancakes) with the optional toasted coconut flakes and enjoy!

9. Alternatively, store the waffles in an airtight container, keep them in the fridge, and consume within 3 days. Store for a maximum of 30 days in the freezer and thaw at room temperature.

Tip: Top the waffles with some Choco Chip Ice Cream with Mint (page 147) or some low-carb fruits like blueberries and sliced strawberries. Cinnamon, vanilla extract, and stevia can be substituted with dry herbs like thyme, rosemary, and/or parsley.

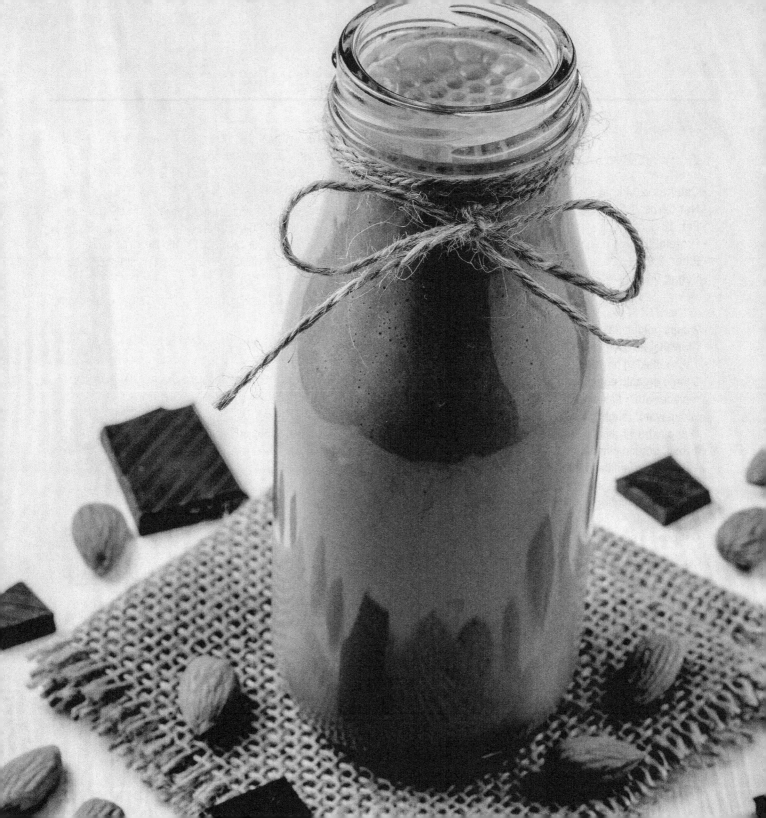

1. Chocolate-Vanilla Almond Milk

Nutrition Information
(per serving)
- Calories: 422 kcal
- Net Carbs: 1.3 g.
- Fat: 34.8 g.
- Protein: 25.5 g.
- Fiber: 2.7 g.
- Sugar: 0.8 g.

INGREDIENTS:
- 2 tbsp. coconut oil
- 1½ cups unsweetened almond milk
- ½ vanilla stick (crushed)
- 1 scoop organic soy protein powder (chocolate flavor)
- 4-6 drops stevia sweetener
- Optional: ½ tsp. cinnamon
- Optional: 1-2 ice cubes

Total number of ingredients: 7

METHOD:
1. Add all the listed ingredients to a blender—except the ice—but including the optional cinnamon if desired.
2. Blend the ingredients for 1 minute; then if desired, add the optional ice cubes and blend for another 30 seconds.
3. Transfer the milk to a large cup or shaker, top with some additional cinnamon, serve, and enjoy!
4. Alternatively, store the smoothie in an airtight container or a mason jar, keep it in the fridge, and consume within 3 days. Store for a maximum of 30 days in the freezer and thaw at room temperature.

SMOOTHIES

2. Nutty Protein Shake 🌿

Serves: 1 | Prep Time: ~5 min |

Nutrition Information
(per serving)
- Calories: 618 kcal
- Net Carbs: 4.4 g.
- Fat: 51.3 g.
- Protein: 34 g.
- Fiber: 4.9 g.
- Sugar: 3 g.

INGREDIENTS:
- 2 tbsp. coconut oil
- 2 cups unsweetened almond milk
- 2 tbsp. peanut butter
- 1 scoop organic soy protein powder
  (chocolate flavor)
- 2-4 ice cubes
- 4-6 drops stevia sweetener
- Optional: 1 tsp. vegan creamer
- Optional: 1 tsp. cocoa powder

Total number of ingredients: 8

METHOD:

1. Add all the above listed ingredients—except the optional ingredients—to a blender, and blend for 2 minutes.

2. Transfer the shake to a large cup or shaker. If desired, top the shake with the optional vegan creamer and/or cocoa powder.

3. Stir before serving, and enjoy!

4. Alternatively, store the smoothie in an airtight container or a mason jar, keep it in the fridge, and consume within 3 days. Store for a maximum of 30 days in the freezer and thaw at room temperature.

3. Chia & Coco Shake 🌱

Nutrition Information
(per serving)
- Calories: 509 kcal
- Net Carbs: 5.4 g.
- Fat: 44.55 g.
- Protein: 20.3 g.
- Fiber: 7.45 g.
- Sugar: 3.5 g.

INGREDIENTS:
- 1 tbsp. chia seeds
- 6 tbsp. water
- 1 cup full-fat coconut milk
- 2 tbsp. peanut butter
- 1 tbsp. MCT oil (or coconut oil)
- 1 scoop organic soy protein powder (chocolate flavor)
- Pinch of Himalayan salt
- 2-4 ice cubes or ½ cup of water

Total number of ingredients: 8

METHOD:
1. Mix the chia seeds and 6 tablespoons of water in a small bowl; let sit for at least 30 minutes.
2. Transfer the soaked chia seeds and all other listed ingredients to a blender and blend for 2 minutes.
3. Transfer the shake to a large cup or shaker, serve, and enjoy!
4. Alternatively, store the smoothie in an airtight container or a mason jar, keep it in the fridge, and consume within 3 days. Store for a maximum of 30 days in the freezer and thaw at room temperature.

Note: This shake will supply you with some additional minerals and electrolytes found in the Himalayan salt!

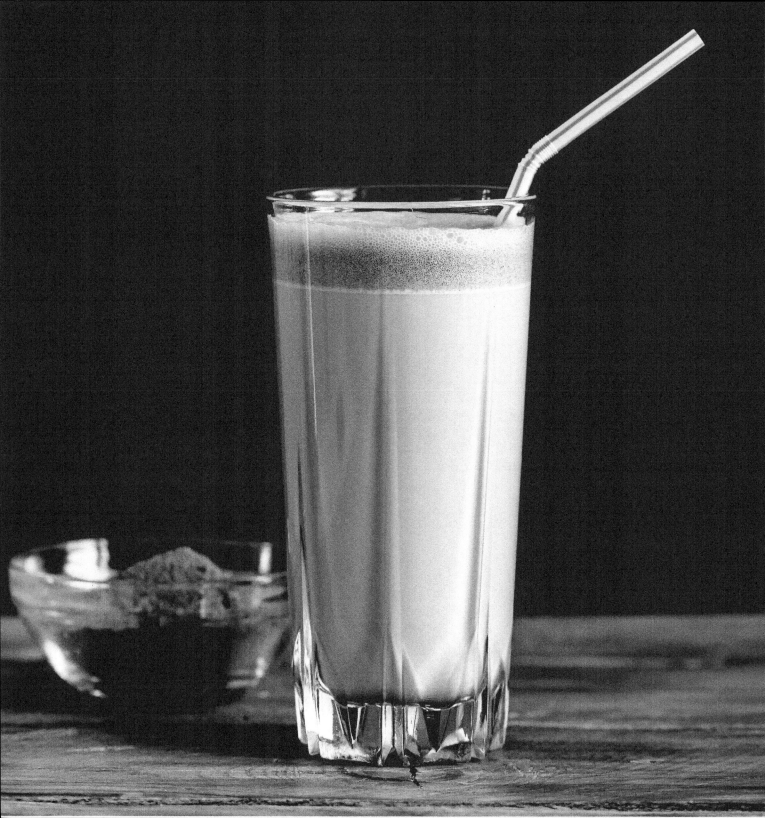

4. Fat-Rich Protein Espresso

Serves: 1 | Prep Time: ~5 min |

Nutrition Information
(per serving)
- Calories: 441 kcal
- Net Carbs: 5.6 g.
- Fat: 34.8 g.
- Protein: 25.4 g.
- Fiber: 6.9 g.
- Sugar: 2.8 g.

INGREDIENTS:

- 1 cup espresso (freshly brewed)
- 2 tbsp. coconut butter
  (or alternatively, use coconut oil)
- 1 scoop organic soy protein
  (chocolate flavor)
- ½ vanilla stick
- 4 ice cubes or ½ cup boiled water
- Optional: 1 tbsp. cacao powder
- Optional: ½ tsp. cinnamon
- 2 tbsp. coconut cream

Total number of ingredients: 8

METHOD:

1. Make sure to use fresh, hot espresso.
2. Add all the listed ingredients to a heat-safe blender, including the ice or boiled water and optional ingredients (if desired). Use ice to make iced espresso, or hot water for a warm treat.
3. Blend the ingredients for 1 minute and transfer to a large coffee cup.
4. Top the coffee with the coconut cream, stir, serve and enjoy!
5. Alternatively, store the smoothie in an airtight container or a mason jar, keep it in the fridge, and consume within 3 days. Store for a maximum of 30 days in the freezer and thaw at room temperature.

Tip: Substitute the coconut cream for a vegan whipping cream or creamer for less fat and a different taste.

5. Raspberry Protein Shake 🍃

Serves: 2 | Prep Time: ~5 min |

Nutrition Information
(per serving)
- Calories: 311 kcal
- Net carbs: 4.6 g.
- Fat: 25.7 g.
- Protein: 14.65 g.
- Fiber: 3.5 g.
- Sugar: 3.35 g.

INGREDIENTS:
- 1 cup full-fat coconut milk
  (or alternatively, use almond milk)
- Optional: ¼ cup coconut cream
- 1 scoop organic soy protein
  (chocolate or vanilla flavor)
- ½ cup raspberries (fresh or frozen)
- 1 tbsp. low-carb maple syrup
- Optional: 2-4 ice cubes

Total number of ingredients: 6

METHOD:
1. Add all the ingredients to a blender, including the optional coconut cream and ice cubes if desired, and blend for 1 minute.

2. Transfer the shake to a large cup or shaker, and enjoy!

3. Alternatively, store the smoothie in an airtight container or a mason jar, keep it in the fridge, and consume within 2 days. Store for a maximum of 30 days in the freezer and thaw at room temperature.

6. Forest Fruit Blaster

Nutrition Information
(per serving)
- Calories: 275 kcal
- Fat:24.8 g.
- Protein: 8.5 g.
- Net carbs: 4 g.
- Fiber: 1.9 g.
- Sugar: 3.4 g.

INGREDIENTS:
- ¼ cup mixed berries (fresh or frozen)
- ½ kiwi (peeled)
- 2 cups full-fat coconut milk
- 2 scoops organic soy protein
  (vanilla flavor)
- ½ cup water
- Optional: 2 ice cubes

Total number of ingredients: 6

METHOD:
1. Add all the ingredients to a blender, including the optional ice if desired, and blend for 1 minute.
2. Transfer the shake to a large cup or shaker, and enjoy!
3. Alternatively, store the smoothie in an airtight container or a mason jar, keep it in the fridge, and consume within 2 days. Store for a maximum of 30 days in the freezer and thaw at room temperature.

7. Vanilla Milkshake

Serves: 1 | Prep Time: ~5 min |

Nutrition Information
(per serving)
- Calories: 600 kcal
- Net carbs: 5.3 g.
- Fat: 46.6 g.
- Protein: 39.3 g.
- Fiber: 4.3 g.
- Sugar: 3.3 g.

INGREDIENTS:
- 2 tbsp. cocoa butter
- 2 cups unsweetened almond milk
- ¼ cup hemp seeds
- 2 tbsp. coconut whipped cream
- 4-6 drops stevia sweetener
- 1 scoop organic soy protein (vanilla flavor)
- 4 ice cubes

Total number of ingredients: 7

METHOD:
1. Add all the ingredients—except the coconut whipped cream—to a blender and blend for 2 minutes.
2. Transfer the shake to a large cup or shaker.
3. Serve with the coconut whipped cream on top, stir, and enjoy!
4. Alternatively, store the smoothie in an airtight container or a mason jar, keep it in the fridge, and consume within 3 days. Store for a maximum of 30 days in the freezer and thaw at room temperature.

Tip: Use another (vegan) whipped cream as a substitute.

8. Raspberry Lemon Protein Smoothie

Nutrition Information
(per serving)
- Calories: 312 kcal
- Net. Carbs: 4.5 g.
- Fat: 27.9 g.
- Protein: 10.15 g.
- Fiber: 4.15 g.
- Sugar: 3 g.

INGREDIENTS:

- ¼ cup flaxseeds
- ½ cup water
- 2 cups full-fat coconut milk
- 1 organic lemon (with peel)
- ½ cup raspberries (fresh or frozen)
- 1 scoop organic soy protein (vanilla flavor)
- 4-6 drops stevia sweetener
- 2 ice cubes

Total number of ingredients: 8

METHOD:

1. Mix the flaxseeds with the water in a medium-sized bowl. Allow the mixture to sit for up to 30 minutes.

2. Add the soaked flaxseeds and the other ingredients to a blender and blend for 2 minutes.

3. Transfer the smoothie to a large cup or shaker, and enjoy!

4. Alternatively, store the smoothie in an airtight container or a mason jar, keep it in the fridge, and consume within 3 days. Store for a maximum of 30 days in the freezer and thaw at room temperature.

9. Breakfast Booster 🌿

Serves: 2 | Prep Time: ~5 min |

Nutrition Information
(per serving)
- Calories: 391 kcal
- Net. Carbs: 4.6 g.
- Fat: 34.65 g.
- Protein: 14.7 g.
- Fiber:2.85 g.
- Sugar: 3.6 g.

INGREDIENTS:
- 1 cup full-fat coconut milk
- 2 tbsp. cocoa butter
- 1 scoop organic soy protein
  (vanilla flavor)
- 4 ice cubes
- Pinch of Himalayan salt
- 5 strawberries (fresh or frozen)
- 1 tsp. matcha powder
- 1 tsp. guarana powder
- 4-6 drops stevia sweetener

Total number of ingredients: 9

METHOD:
1. Add all the required ingredients to a blender and blend for 1 minute.
2. Transfer the shake to a large cup or shaker, and enjoy!
3. Alternatively, store the smoothie in an airtight container or a mason jar, keep it in the fridge, and consume within 2 days. Store for a maximum of 30 days in the freezer and thaw at room temperature.

10. Cinnamon Pear Protein Shake

Serves: 1 | Prep Time: ~5 min |

Nutrition Information
(per serving)
- Calories: 398 kcal
- Net Carbs: 5.4 g.
- Fat: 28 g.
- Protein: 28.8 g.
- Fiber: 14.9 g.
- Sugar: 4.4 g.

INGREDIENTS:
- 1 tsp. freeze-dried pear powder
- 1 medium Hass avocado
  (peeled, pitted, and halved)
- 2 cups unsweetened almond milk
- 1 scoop organic soy protein (vanilla flavor)
- ½ tsp. cinnamon
- 4-6 drops stevia sweetener
- 2 ice cubes

Total number of ingredients: 7

METHOD:
1. Add all the required ingredients to a blender, including the optional ice cubes if desired, and blend for 1 minute.

2. Transfer to a large cup or shaker and enjoy!

3. Alternatively, store the smoothie in an airtight container or a mason jar, keep it in the fridge, and consume within 3 days. Store for a maximum of 30 days in the freezer and thaw at room temperature.

1. Indian Egg Salad

Serves: 2 | Prep Time: ~25 min |

Nutrition Information
(per serving)
- Calories: 510 kcal
- Net Carbs: 6.8 g.
- Fat: 46.8 g.
- Protein: 14 g.
- Fiber: 8.7 g.
- Sugar: 5.3 g.

INGREDIENTS:

- 1 large Hass avocado
  (peeled, pitted, and halved)
- 4 medium organic eggs
- ¼ cup full-fat mayonnaise
- Sea salt and black pepper to taste
- 1 tbsp. fresh lemon juice
- 1 red bell pepper (pitted, diced)
- 1 tsp. dried oregano
- 1 tbsp. curry powder
- 1 tbsp. fresh cilantro (chopped)

Total number of ingredients: 10

METHOD:

1. Put the eggs in a saucepan filled with water. Bring the water to a boil over medium heat.

2. Once the water boils, turn the heat down to low and cover the saucepan. Allow the eggs to sit in simmering water for 6-12 minutes (6 minutes for a soft yolk, and up to 12 minutes for a thoroughly-cooked yolk).

3. Take the saucepan off the heat, drain the hot water, and rinse the eggs with cold water. Peel the eggs and set aside.

4. Put the diced bell pepper in a medium-sized bowl, add the avocado, and mix them together with a masher.

5. Add the cooked eggs, mayonnaise, lemon juice, dried oregano, and curry powder to the bowl.

6. Mash everything together into a spicy egg salad while adding salt and pepper to taste.

7. Garnish the egg salad with freshly chopped cilantro for serving and enjoy!

8. Alternatively, store this in the fridge using an air-tight container and consume within 3 days.

LUNCHES

2. Asparagus and Egg Salad

Serves: 2 | Prep Time: ~20 min |

Nutrition Information
(per serving)
- Calories: 398 kcal
- Net Carbs: 3.9 g.
- Fat: 35.4 g.
- Protein: 15.5 g.
- Fiber: 4.3 g.
- Sugar: 3.5 g.

INGREDIENTS:
- 10 asparagus spears
- 3 large organic eggs
- ¼ cup pine nuts
- 1 tbsp. apple cider vinegar
- 2 tbsp. olive oil
- ¼ cup fresh lovage (chopped)
- ½ tbsp. dried thyme
- Sea salt and black pepper to taste

Total number of ingredients: 9

METHOD:
1. Put the eggs in a saucepan filled with water. Bring the water to a boil over medium heat.

2. Once the water boils, turn the heat down to low and cover the saucepan. Allow the eggs to sit in simmering water for 6-12 minutes (6 minutes for a soft yolk and up to 12 minutes for a thoroughly-cooked yolk).

3. Take the saucepan off the heat, drain the hot water, and rinse the eggs with cold water. Peel the eggs and set aside.

4. Cook the asparagus with 1 tablespoon of olive oil in a frying pan over high heat for about 2 minutes. Make sure to turn the asparagus occasionally until they are tender.

5. Take the pan off the heat and chop the asparagus into ½-inch pieces. Set aside.

6. Cut the peeled eggs in half, mash the yolks and egg whites in two separate small bowls, and season both with salt and pepper to taste.

7. Use a large salad bowl to mix the apple cider vinegar with 1 tablespoon of olive oil. Add salt and pepper to taste.

8. Add the cooked asparagus, egg mixtures, thyme, and chopped lovage to the salad bowl.

9. Toss the ingredients to mix everything together. Then serve the salad topped with the pine nuts, and enjoy!

10. Alternatively, store it in the fridge using an airtight container and consume within 2 days.

Note: If storing, separate (store separately) the pine nuts and the salad; top the salad just before serving.

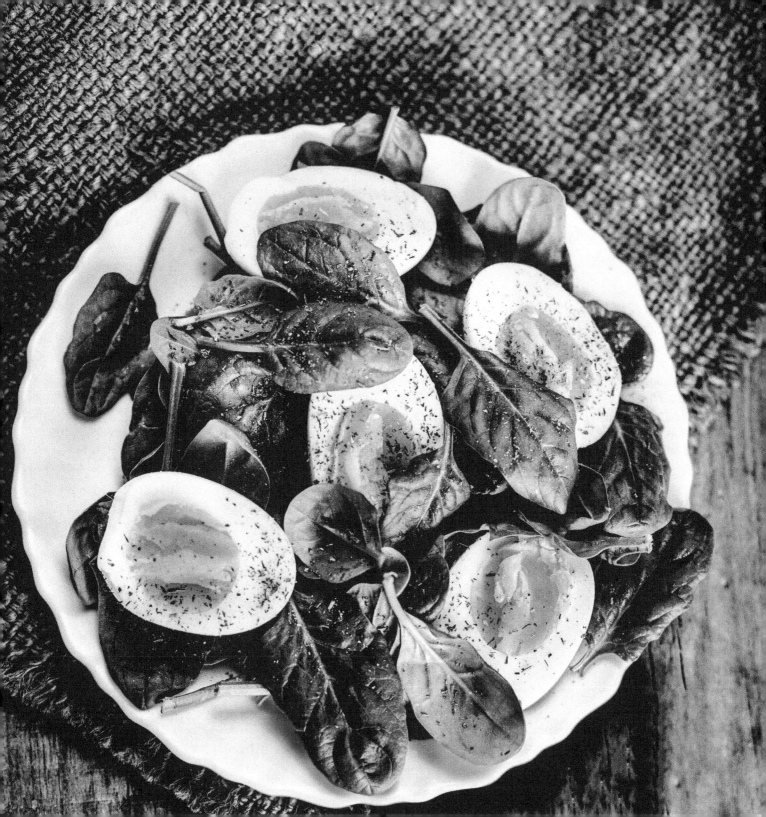

3. Eggs and Spinach Salad 🥚

Serves: 2 | Prep Time: ~25 min |

Nutrition Information
(per serving)
- Calories: 275 kcal
- Net Carbs: 4.7 g.
- Fat: 22.2 g.
- Protein: 13.7 g.
- Fiber: 1.8 g.
- Sugar: 2.9 g.

INGREDIENTS:
- 4 medium organic eggs
- 4 cups baby spinach leaves
  (rinsed and drained)
- 2 medium shallots (finely minced)
- 1 tbsp. lemon juice
- 1½ tbsp. olive oil
- Sea salt and black pepper to taste

Total number of ingredients: 7

METHOD:
1. Put the eggs in a saucepan filled with water. Bring the water to a boil over medium heat.
2. Once the water boils, turn the heat down to low and cover the saucepan. Allow the eggs to sit in simmering water for 6-12 minutes (6 minutes for a soft yolk, and up to 12 minutes for a thoroughly-cooked yolk).
3. Take the saucepan off the heat, drain the hot water, and rinse the eggs with cold water. Peel the eggs and set aside.
4. Transfer the eggs to a medium bowl and add the lemon juice, 1 tablespoon of olive oil, minced shallots, and salt and pepper to taste.
5. Mash everything together with a potato masher into a chunky egg salad.
6. Serve the salad over a bed of baby spinach leaves, and sprinkle it with half a tablespoon of olive oil.
7. Toss the salad to mix everything together, serve, and enjoy!
8. Alternatively, store it in the fridge using an airtight container and consume within 2 days.

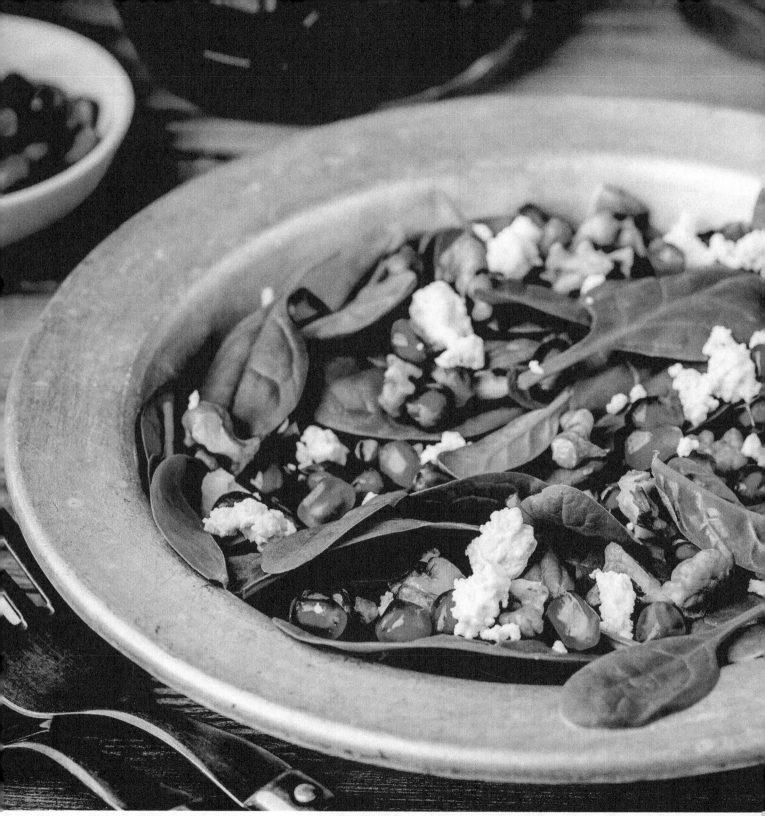

4. Spinach and Feta Salad

Nutrition Information
(per serving)
- Calories: 504 kcal
- Net Carbs: 7.7 g.
- Fat: 45.8 g.
- Protein: 15.1 g.
- Fiber: 2.1 g.
- Sugar: 4.2 g.

INGREDIENTS:

- 6 cups baby spinach leaves
  (rinsed and drained)
- 2 cups feta cheese (cubed)
- ½ cup walnuts
- 1 tbsp. low-carb maple syrup
- 1 garlic clove (finely minced)
- 2 tbsp. fresh lemon juice
- 2 tbsp. olive oil
- Sea salt and black pepper to taste
- Optional: ¼ cup pomegranate seeds

Total number of ingredients: 10

METHOD:

1. Take a medium-sized bowl and mix in the lemon juice, maple syrup, and olive oil with salt and pepper to taste.

2. Add the minced garlic to the lemon juice dressing, and mix the ingredients thoroughly. Set aside.

3. Put the spinach in a large salad bowl, add the feta cheese, and toss well to mix everything together.

4. Add the lemon juice dressing, toss the salad again, and mix in the walnuts.

5. Add more salt and pepper to taste.

6. Serve the salad—topped with optional pomegranate seeds if desired—and enjoy!

7. Alternatively, store it in the fridge using an airtight container and consume within 2 days.

5. Fried Halloumi and Egg Scramble

Serves: 2 | Prep Time: ~20 min |

Nutrition Information
(per serving)
- Calories: 627 kcal
- Net Carbs: 8.6 g.
- Fat: 52.2 g.
- Protein: 29.4 g.
- Fiber: 9.3 g.
- Sugar: 6.2 g.

INGREDIENTS:
- 1 large Hass avocado
  (peeled, pitted, and sliced)
- 4 medium organic eggs
- 1 cup halloumi cheese (cubed)
- 1 shallot (finely minced)
- 1 garlic clove (finely minced)
- ¼ cup fresh lovage (chopped)
- 1 tbsp. dried oregano
- 10 black olives
- 2 tbsp. olive oil
- Sea salt and black pepper to taste
- 2 tbsp. fresh lemon juice
- Optional: ¼ cup pine nuts

Total number of ingredients: 13

METHOD:

1. Put a large skillet over medium-high heat and add olive oil, shallot, and garlic.

2. Add the halloumi to the skillet and stir-fry the ingredients until they are browned nicely.

3. Take a medium-sized bowl and mix in the eggs, lovage, and oregano. Add salt and pepper to taste.

4. Stir the egg mixture and then transfer it to the skillet. Lower the heat to medium-low.

5. Stir in the avocado slices and olives, and continue to stir until the eggs are scrambled.

6. Drizzle the lemon juice over the egg scramble, top with the optional pine nuts (if desired), serve, and enjoy!

7. Alternatively, store the egg scramble in the fridge, using an airtight container, and consume within 3 days. Store in the freezer for a maximum of 30 days, and thaw at room temperature. Use a microwave, toaster oven, or pan to reheat the egg scramble.

Note: If storing, separate (i.e., store separately) the pine nuts, lemon juice, and scramble; top right before serving.

6. Deviled Red Pepper Eggs

Serves: 3 | Prep Time: ~25 min |

Nutrition Information
(per serving)
- Calories: 176 kcal
- Net Carbs: 5.7 g.
- Fat: 10.6 g.
- Protein: 14 g.
- Fiber: 3 g.
- Sugar: 4.5 g.

INGREDIENTS:
- 6 large organic eggs
- 1 small Ramiro pepper
- 1 shallot (finely minced)
- ½ tbsp. mango chutney
- Optional: 1-2 tbsp. water
- 1 tbsp. smoked paprika powder
- 1 tbsp. curry powder
- 1 tsp. ginger powder
- 2 tbsp. chives (finely minced)

Total number of ingredients: 9

METHOD:

1. Put the eggs in a saucepan filled with water. Bring the water to a boil over medium heat.

2. Once the water boils, turn the heat down to low and cover the saucepan. Allow the eggs to sit in simmering water for 6-12 minutes (6 minutes for a soft yolk, and up to 12 minutes for a thoroughly-cooked yolk).

3. Take the saucepan off the heat, drain the hot water, and rinse the eggs with cold water. Peel the eggs and cut them in half. Take out the yolks and transfer these to a medium bowl. Set the bowl and the halved egg whites aside.

4. Slice the Ramiro pepper in half lengthwise; remove the seeds, stem, and placenta and discard. Slice the pepper into tiny cubes.

5. Add the Ramiro pepper cubes, minced shallot, mango chutney, paprika powder, curry powder, and ginger powder to the bowl with the egg yolks. For a more liquid consistency, blend in the optional water.

6. Mash all the ingredients together until it is thoroughly mixed.

7. Fill each halved egg white with teaspoons of the yolk mixture until no yolk mixture is left.

8. Top the eggs with some finely minced chives, serve, and enjoy!

9. Alternatively, store the deviled eggs in an airtight container, keep them in the fridge, and consume within 3 days.

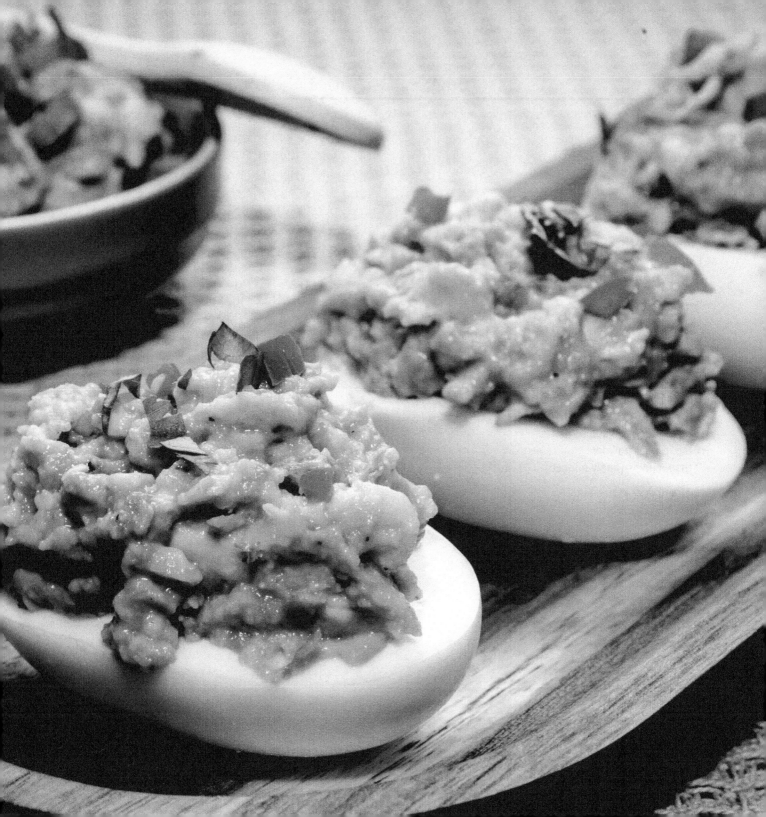

7. Guacamole-Filled Eggs

Serves: 3 | Prep Time: ~25 min |

Nutrition Information
(per serving)
- Calories: 180 kcal
- Net Carbs: 2.5 g.
- Fat: 13 g.
- Protein: 13.1 g.
- Fiber: 1.9 g.
- Sugar: 1.5 g.

INGREDIENTS:
- 6 large organic eggs
- ½ small Hass avocado (peeled and pitted)
- 1 tsp. Dijon mustard
- 1 small garlic clove (finely minced)
- 1 tsp. sugar-free pickle juice
- Pinch of sea salt and black pepper
- ½ tsp. sugar
- 1 tbsp. fresh cilantro (finely chopped)

Total number of ingredients: 9

METHOD:
1. Put the eggs in a saucepan filled with water. Bring the water to a boil over medium heat.

2. Once the water boils, turn the heat down to low, and cover the saucepan. Allow the eggs to sit in simmering water for 6-12 minutes (6 minutes for a soft yolk, and up to 12 minutes for a thoroughly-cooked yolk).

3. Take the saucepan off the heat, drain the hot water, and rinse the eggs with cold water. Peel the eggs and cut them in half. Take out the yolks and transfer these to a medium bowl. Set the bowl and the halved egg whites aside.

4. Scoop out the avocado half and add it to the bowl with egg yolks.

5. Add the remaining ingredients—except the cilantro—to the bowl and mash everything together until it is thoroughly mixed.

6. Fill each egg white with a tablespoon of the yolk mixture.

7. Top the eggs with some finely minced cilantro, serve, and enjoy!

8. Alternatively, store the filled eggs in an airtight container, keep them in the fridge, and consume within 3 days.

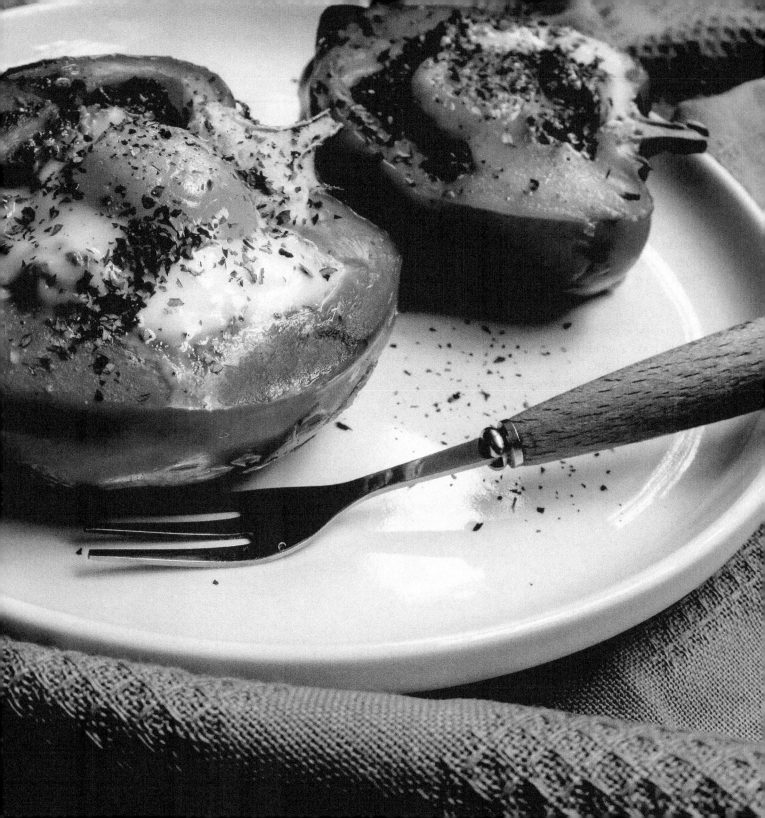

8. Egg-Stuffed Bell Peppers

Serves: 3 | Prep Time: ~40 min |

Nutrition Information
(per serving)
- Calories: 348 kcal
- Net Carbs: 8.1 g.
- Fat: 27 g.
- Protein: 16.2 g.
- Fiber: 11.6 g.
- Sugar: 5.7 g.

INGREDIENTS:

- 6 large organic eggs
- 3 bell peppers
  (red or yellow—halved and seeded)
- 2 medium Hass avocados
  (peeled, pitted, and halved)
- 1 cup tomatoes (skinned and cubed)
- ¼ cup red onion (minced)
- 2 jalapenos
- 4 tbsp. lime juice
- 1 tbsp. smoked paprika powder
- 1 garlic clove (minced)
- 1 tsp. ground cumin seeds
- 1 tsp. dried oregano
- Pinch of Himalayan salt
- ¼ cup fresh cilantro (chopped)

Total number of ingredients: 13

METHOD:

1. Preheat oven to 375°F / 190°C, and line a baking sheet with parchment paper.

2. Take a large bowl, crack the eggs in it, and whisk. Add salt and pepper to taste.

3. Halve the jalapenos; remove the stems, seeds, and placenta, and discard. Chop jalapenos into tiny pieces.

4. Add the avocados to the bowl with eggs, along with 2 tablespoons of lime juice, tomato, jalapenos, red onion, salt, and remaining spices except the cilantro.

5. Mix everything with a potato masher until thoroughly combined.

6. Fill the bell pepper halves with tablespoons of the egg mixture. Divide the mixture equally.

7. Transfer the 6 stuffed bell pepper halves to the baking sheet. Bake them for 25-30 minutes.

8. Take the tray out; sprinkle the stuffed bell pepper halves with the remaining lime juice and chopped cilantro, serve, and enjoy.

9. Alternatively, store the bell peppers in the fridge, using an airtight container and consume within 3 days. Store in the freezer for a maximum of 30 days and thaw at room temperature. Use a microwave or toaster oven to reheat the bell peppers.

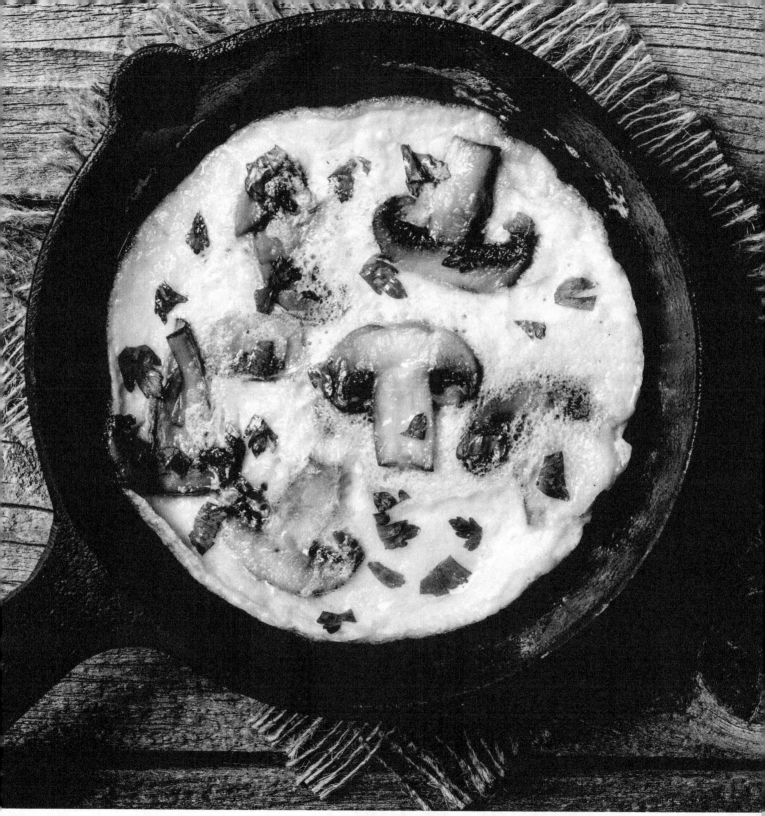

9. Mushroom Duo Omelet

Nutrition Information
(per serving)
- Calories: 377 kcal
- Net Carbs: 5.9 g.
- Fat: 28.3 g.
- Protein: 24.1 g.
- Fiber: 3.7 g.
- Sugar: 3.8 g.

INGREDIENTS:

- 3 large organic eggs
- ½ tsp. fresh thyme (chopped)
- 1 tbsp. extra virgin olive oil
- ½ cup button mushrooms (sliced)
- ¼ cup portabella mushrooms (sliced)
- ¼ cup yellow onions (diced)
- Sea salt and ground black pepper to taste
- 1 tsp. fresh parsley (chopped)

Total number of ingredients: 9

METHOD:

1. Crack the eggs into a medium bowl and use a whisk to incorporate the yolks with the egg whites.

2. Add the thyme, salt, and pepper to the egg mixture. Use the whisk to incorporate all ingredients.

3. Place a medium-sized skillet over medium-high heat and add the olive oil.

4. Add the sliced mushrooms and diced onions to the skillet. Sauté the vegetables while stirring until they are soft and tender.

5. Once the vegetables are sautéed, add the egg mixture to the skillet. Cook the omelet for about 5 minutes, until the omelet begins to firm up.

6. Carefully run a spatula around the edge of the pan. If the omelet need to cook a little longer, flip it over and cook the other side for no more than 1 minute.

7. Fold the omelet in half with the spatula and transfer it to a plate.

8. Serve the omelet with freshly chopped parsley and additional spices, and enjoy!

9. Alternatively, store the omelet in an airtight container the fridge, and consume within 3 days. Store in the freezer for a maximum of 30 days and thaw at room temperature. Use a microwave, toaster oven, or pan to reheat the omelet.

Tip: The yellow onions can be combined with green onions.

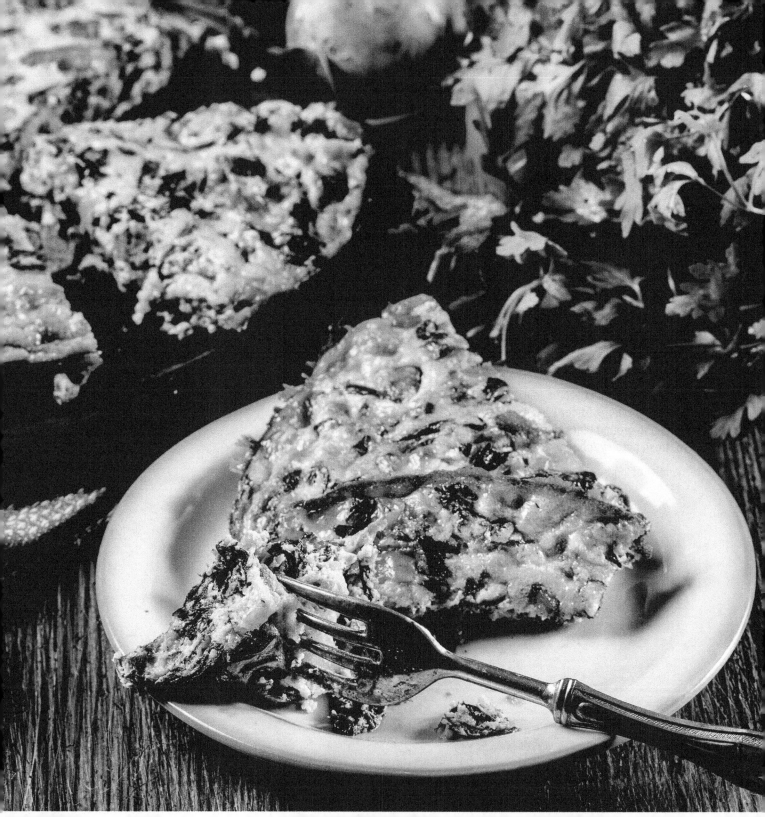

10. Avocado and Cauliflower Hummus

Serves: 2 | Prep Time: ~20 min |

Nutrition Information
(per serving)
- Calories: 416 kcal
- Net Carbs: 8.4 g.
- Fat: 40.3 g.
- Protein: 3.3 g.
- Fiber: 10.3 g.
- Sugar: 7.1 g.

INGREDIENTS:
- 1 medium cauliflower
  (stem removed and chopped)
- 1 large Hass avocado
  (peeled, pitted, and chopped)
- ¼ cup extra virgin olive oil
- 2 small garlic cloves
- ½ tbsp. lemon juice
- ½ tsp. onion powder
- Sea salt and ground black pepper to taste
- 2 large carrots
  (peeled and cut into fries,
  or use store-bought raw carrot fries)
- Optional: ¼ cup fresh cilantro (chopped)

Total number of ingredients: 10

METHOD:
1. Preheat the oven to 450°F / 220°C, and line a baking tray with aluminum foil.
2. Put the chopped cauliflower on the baking tray and drizzle with 2 tablespoons of olive oil.
3. Roast the chopped cauliflower in the oven for 20-25 minutes, until lightly brown.
4. Remove the tray from the oven and allow the cauliflower to cool down.
5. Add all the ingredients—except the carrots and optional fresh cilantro—to a food processor or blender, and blend the ingredients into a smooth hummus.
6. Transfer the hummus to a medium-sized bowl, cover, and put it in the fridge for at least 30 minutes.
7. Take the hummus out of the fridge and, if desired, top it with the optional chopped cilantro and more salt and pepper to taste; serve with the carrot fries, and enjoy!
8. Alternatively, store it in the fridge in an airtight container, and consume within 2 days.

Tip: For baked fries, bake the carrot slices in the oven with olive oil, salt, and pepper at 450°F / 220°C for 15-20 minutes. This hummus can also be served on top of the bread from Tofu Stir-Fry on Almond Bread (page 132).

11. Full-Fat Egg Salad

Nutrition Information
(per serving)
- Calories: 338 kcal
- Net Carbs: 1.7g.
- Fat: 32.2g.
- Protein: 10g.
- Fiber: 2.5g.
- Sugar: 0.9g.

INGREDIENTS:
- 1 large Hass avocado
  (peeled, pitted, and sliced)
- 6 large organic eggs
  (boiled and peeled)
- ½ cup full-fat mayonnaise
- 1 tbsp. lemon juice
- 1 tbsp. fresh parsley (chopped)
- 1 tsp. Dijon mustard
- Sea salt and black pepper to taste

Total number of ingredients: 8

METHOD:

1. Put the eggs in a saucepan filled with water. Bring the water to a boil over medium heat.

2. Once the water boils, turn the heat down to low and cover the saucepan. Allow the eggs to sit in simmering water for 6-12 minutes (6 minutes for a soft yolk, and up to 12 minutes for a thoroughly-cooked yolk).

3. Take the saucepan off the heat, drain the hot water, and rinse the eggs with cold water. Peel the eggs and transfer them to a large bowl.

4. Chop the eggs into small chunks, add the avocado slices, and mash both ingredients with a fork. Top the mixture with salt and pepper to taste.

5. Add all the remaining ingredients and mash them together with a fork.

6. Top the salad with some additional salt and pepper to taste.

7. Give the salad another stir and then transfer the bowl to the fridge.

8. Chill the egg salad for at least 1 hour before serving, and then enjoy!

9. Alternatively, store the salad in the fridge, using an airtight container and consume within 3 days.

Tip: Add more mayonnaise or eggs if desired. Serve this mixture with the Protein Nut 'N Seed Bread (page 41)!

12. Goat Cheese Salad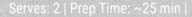

Serves: 2 | Prep Time: ~25 min |

Nutrition Information
(per serving)
- Calories: 704 kcal
- Net Carbs: 6.8 g.
- Fat: 59 g.
- Protein: 37.6 g.
- Fiber: 3.2 g.
- Sugar: 4.6 g.

INGREDIENTS:
- 1½ cups goat cheese (soft and sliced)
- ¼ cup roasted pumpkin seeds
- ¼ cup grass-fed butter
- 1 tbsp. balsamic vinegar
- 3 cups fresh spinach leaves (chopped)
- 12 cherry tomatoes (halved)
- 1 tsp. dried oregano

Total number of ingredients: 7

METHOD:

1. Preheat oven to 400°F / 200°C, and grease a baking dish with ½ tablespoon of butter.

2. Put the sliced goat cheese in the dish and heat it in the oven for 10 minutes.

3. Meanwhile, put a medium-sized skillet over medium heat and add the roasted pumpkin seeds and the rest of the butter while constantly stirring.

4. Add the vinegar and allow the mixture in the skillet to boil for a minute before turning off the heat.

5. Spread the spinach leaves on 2 plates, and top with the molten cheese from the baking tray. Then cover it with the butter mixture from the skillet.

6. Serve the salad with the cherry tomatoes and dried oregano on top, and enjoy!

7. Alternatively, store the salad in the fridge using an airtight container, and consume within 2 days.

Tip: Use different types of goat cheeses for a different flavor—a soft type for the oven, and a harder type to crumble on top of the salad.

13. Veggie Supreme Omelet

Serves: 1 | Prep Time: ~15 min |

Nutrition Information
(per serving)
- Calories: 375 kcal
- Net Carbs: 7 g.
- Fat: 28.1 g.
- Protein: 23.1 g.
- Fiber: 3.6 g.
- Sugar: 4 g.

INGREDIENTS:
- 3 large organic eggs
- ½ cup fresh spinach (chopped)
- ½ tsp. garlic powder
- 1 tbsp. extra virgin olive oil
- ½ cup button mushrooms (sliced)
- ¼ cup red bell pepper (pitted and diced)
- ¼ cup yellow onions (diced)
- 1 tsp. fresh parsley (chopped)
- Kosher salt and ground black pepper to taste

Total number of ingredients: 10

METHOD:
1. Crack the eggs into a medium-sized bowl and use a whisk to incorporate the yolks with the egg whites.
2. Add the spinach, garlic powder, salt, and pepper to taste. Use the whisk to incorporate all ingredients into a smooth mixture.
3. Place a medium-sized skillet over medium-high heat and add the olive oil.
4. Add the mushrooms, red bell peppers, and onions to the skillet. Sauté the vegetables until they are soft and tender. Stir occasionally to prevent the vegetables from sticking to the pan or burning.
5. Once the vegetables are sautéed, add the egg mixture to the skillet. Cook the mixture for about 5 minutes until the omelet begins to firm up.
6. Carefully run the spatula around the edge of the pan. If the omelet needs to cook a little longer, flip it over and cook the other side for no more than 1 minute.
7. Fold the omelet in half and transfer it to a plate.
8. Serve the omelet with freshly chopped parsley and enjoy!
9. Alternatively, store the omelet in the fridge, using an airtight container, and consume within 3 days. Store in the freezer for a maximum of 30 days and thaw at room temperature. Use a microwave, toaster oven, or pan to reheat the omelet.

Tip: Add more leafy greens to this omelet and substitute the red bell pepper for a yellow version.

14. Feta Salad with Scrambled Tofu 🥛

Serves: 4 | Prep Time: ~25 min |

Nutrition Information
(per serving)
- Calories: 421 kcal
- Net Carbs: 6.1 g.
- Fat: 37.8 g.
- Protein: 13.9 g.
- Fiber: 1.6 g.
- Sugar: 4.2 g.

INGREDIENTS:

Salad:
- 1 8-oz. pack firm tofu (drained and cubed)
- 1½ tbsp. olive oil
- 5 medium sundried tomatoes (chopped)
- ½ cucumber (chopped)
- 1½ cups feta cheese (crumbled)
- ½ medium green onion (sliced)
- 10 black olives (pitted)
- Optional: 4 tbsp. roasted pumpkin pits

Dressing:
- 5 tbsp. olive oil
- 1 tbsp. red wine vinegar
- 1 tsp. dried oregano
- ½ tsp. garlic powder
  (alternatively, use 1 minced garlic clove)
- Optional: salt and black pepper to taste

Total number of ingredients: 14

METHOD:

1. Take a medium-sized skillet and put it over medium heat.
2. Add 1 tablespoon of olive oil and the tofu cubes. Crush the tofu with a wooden spatula while stirring.
3. Cook the tofu crumbles for up to 6 minutes, until they start to brown. Then take the skillet off the heat and set the tofu aside.
4. Take a large bowl and add the tomatoes, cucumber, feta, and onions.
5. Toss the ingredients and add the olives and, if desired, the optional pumpkin pits.
6. Take a separate small bowl and mix in all the dressing ingredients; add salt and black pepper to taste.
7. Make sure all salad ingredients are mixed well, top it with the dressing, serve, and enjoy!
8. Alternatively, store the salad in the fridge using an airtight container, and consume within 3 days.

Note: Leave the tofu out for a soy-free salad!

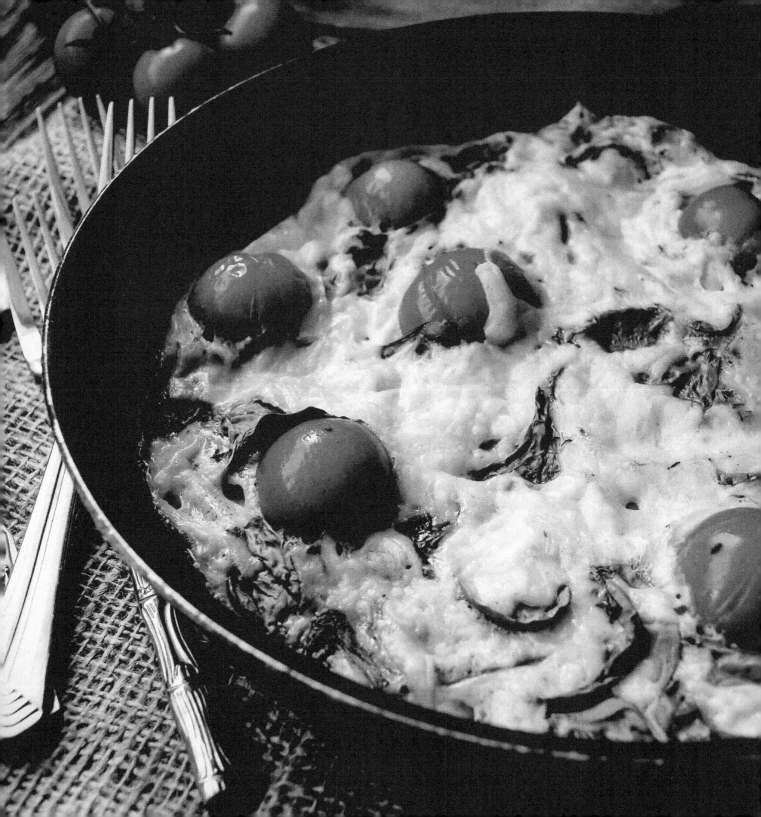

15. Keto Southwestern Omelet

Serves: 1 | Prep Time: ~15 min |

Nutrition Information
(per serving)
- Calories: 364 kcal
- Net Carbs: 5 g.
- Fat: 28.9 g.
- Protein: 20.6 g.
- Fiber: 3.3 g.
- Sugar: 1.9 g.

INGREDIENTS:
- 3 large organic eggs
- ½ tsp. fresh parsley (chopped)
- ½ cup fresh spinach (chopped)
- 1 tsp. chili powder
- 1 tbsp. extra virgin olive oil
- ¼ cup yellow onion (diced)
- ¼ cup cherry tomatoes (sliced)
- Optional: ¼ cup canned black beans (drained)
- 1 tsp. fresh parsley (chopped)
- Kosher salt and ground black pepper to taste

Total number of ingredients: 11

METHOD:

1. Crack the eggs into a medium-sized bowl and use a whisk to incorporate the yolks with the egg whites.

2. Add the parsley, spinach, chili powder, salt, and pepper to taste. Use the whisk to incorporate all ingredients.

3. Place a medium-sized skillet over medium-high heat and add the olive oil.

4. Add the onions to the skillet and sauté until soft and tender, about 3 minutes.

5. Stir in the cherry tomatoes and, if desired, the optional black beans. Heat the ingredients for an additional 2 minutes.

6. Add the egg mixture to the skillet. Stir and cook the omelet for about 5 minutes, until it begins to firm up.

7. Carefully run a spatula around the edge of the pan to release the omelet. Flip the omelet over and cook the other side for no more than 1 minute.

8. Fold the omelet in half and transfer it to a plate.

9. Serve the omelet with freshly chopped parsley and enjoy!

10. Alternatively, store the omelet in the fridge in an airtight container, and consume within 3 days. Store in the freezer for a maximum of 30 days and thaw at room temperature. Use a microwave, toaster oven or pan to reheat the omelet.

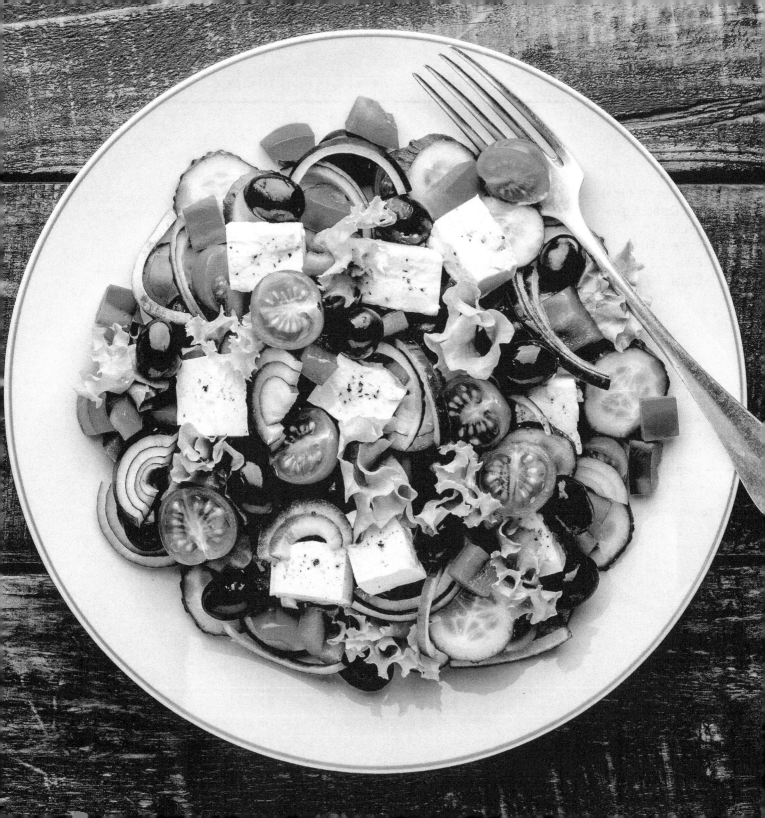

16. Greek Feta Salad

Nutrition Information
(per serving)
- Calories: 506 kcal
- Net Carbs: 10.2 g.
- Fat: 45.8 g.
- Protein: 12.7 g.
- Fiber: 3.9 g.
- Sugar: 7.3 g.

INGREDIENTS:

- 2 tbsp. extra virgin olive oil
- 2 tbsp. red wine vinegar
- ½ tsp. dried oregano
- ½ tsp. garlic powder
- 1 cup red leaf lettuce (chopped)
- ½ cup tomatoes (diced)
- ¼ cup red onions (sliced)
- ½ cup cucumbers (sliced into half-moons)
- ½ cup Feta cheese (crumbled)
- 5 Kalamata or black olives (halved)
- Kosher salt and ground black pepper to taste

Total number of ingredients: 12

METHOD:

1. Take a small bowl and add 1 tablespoon of olive oil, the red wine vinegar, dried oregano, salt, pepper, and garlic powder. Combine all ingredients together with a whisk.

2. Add the chopped lettuce, tomatoes, red onions, and cucumbers to separate large bowl. Mix and toss the ingredients well.

3. Give the dressing in the small bowl one more stir, and then divide it over the mixed vegetables.

4. Continue to toss the salad until the ingredients are completely coated.

5. Top the salad with the Feta cheese and olives.

6. Add 1 more tablespoon of olive oil, toss again, serve, and enjoy!

7. Alternatively, store the salad in the fridge using an airtight container and consume within 2 days.

Tip: Add some scrambled tofu to increase the protein in this salad.

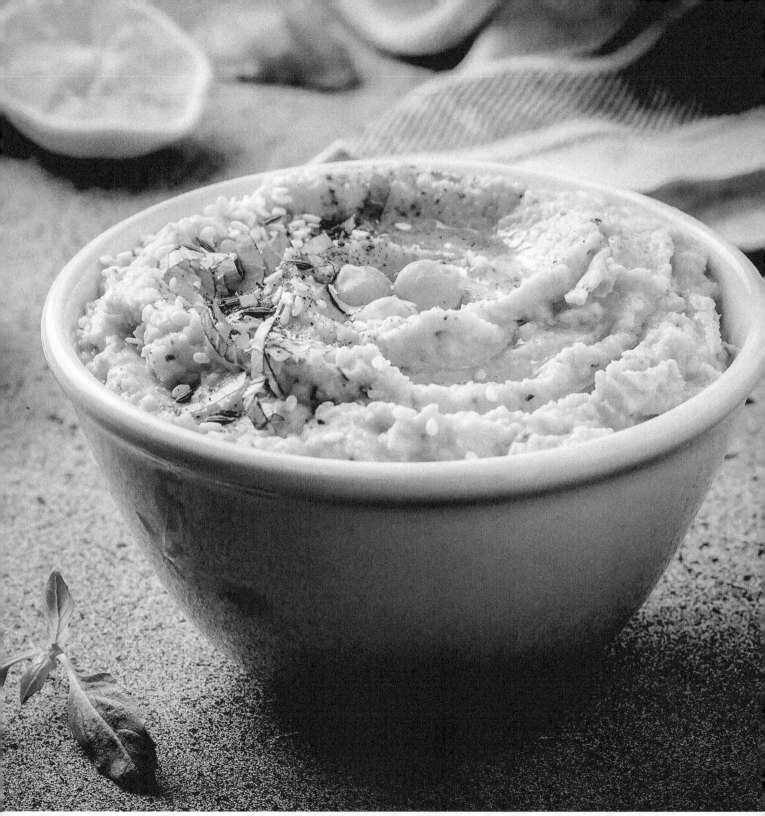

17. Caprese Salad

Serves: 4 | Prep Time: ~15 min |

Nutrition Information
(per serving)
- Calories: 471 kcal
- Net Carbs: 4.4 g.
- Fat: 44.4 g.
- Protein: 13.5 g.
- Fiber: 3 g.
- Sugar: 3.0 g.

INGREDIENTS:

Macadamia Pesto:
- ⅓ cup raw macadamia nuts
- 2 cups fresh basil
- ⅓ cup parmesan cheese (grated)
- 4 tbsp. olive oil
- 3 small garlic cloves (minced)
- Sea salt and black pepper to taste

Salad:
- ⅔ cup mozzarella cheese (sliced)
- 4 cups lettuce leaves (chopped)
- 3 tbsp. olive oil
- 5 tbsp. hemp seeds
- 1 tbsp. nutritional yeast
- 1 tsp. cayenne pepper

Total number of ingredients: 13

METHOD:

1. Add the macadamia nuts to a blender or food processor. Pulse the nuts into small pieces before adding the remaining macadamia pesto ingredients.

2. Blend the ingredients into a smooth pesto mixture with some small chunks left in it. Scraping the sides of the blender with a spatula will help to incorporate all ingredients.

3. Transfer the pesto to a medium-sized bowl and refrigerate it for up to 1 hour.

4. Heat up a medium-sized skillet over medium heat and add 3 tablespoons of olive oil.

5. Add the hemp seeds while stirring.

6. Toast the seeds for 5 minutes, then add the nutritional yeast. Stir and toast for another 5 minutes and turn off the heat. Set the skillet aside.

7. Fill a large bowl with the chopped lettuce, macadamia pesto, and mozzarella slices.

8. Top with the toasted hemp seeds, add cayenne pepper before serving, and enjoy!

9. Alternatively, store the salad in the fridge using an airtight container and consume within 2 days.

Tip: Toast the hemp seeds with a different oil for another flavor. The mozzarella can be substituted or mixed with boiled egg whites.

18. Raw Zoodles with Avocado 'N Nuts ❦

Serves: 2 | Prep Time: ~10 min |

Nutrition Information
(per serving)
- Calories: 317 kcal
- Net Carbs: 7.4 g.
- Fat: 28.1 g.
- Protein: 7.2 g.
- Fiber: 8.9 g.
- Sugar: 5.6 g.

INGREDIENTS:
- 1 medium zucchini
  (spiralized into zoodles
  or sliced into very thin slices)
- 1½ cups basil
- ⅓ cup water
- 5 tbsp. pine nuts
- 2 tbsp. lemon juice
- 1 medium avocado
  (peeled, pitted, and sliced)
- Optional: 2 tbsp. olive oil
- 6 yellow cherry tomatoes (halved)
- Optional: 6 red cherry tomatoes (halved)
- Sea salt and black pepper to taste

Total number of ingredients: 11

METHOD:
1. Add the basil, water, nuts, lemon juice, avocado slices, optional olive oil (if desired), salt, and pepper to a blender.

2. Blend the ingredients into a smooth mixture. Add more salt and pepper to taste and blend again.

3. Divide the sauce and the zucchini noodles between two medium-sized bowls for serving, and combine in each.

4. Top the mixtures with the halved yellow cherry tomatoes, and the optional red cherry tomatoes (if desired); serve and enjoy!

5. Alternatively, store the zoodles in the fridge using an airtight container and consume within 2 days.

Tip: Add more spiralized or sliced veggies—like cabbage—to add flavor. The salad can be topped with additional nuts, seeds, or more oil.

1. Mozzarella Cheese 🌿

Serves: 16 / 1 block of cheese | Prep Time: ~20 min |

Nutrition Information
(per serving)
- Calories: 101 kcal
- Net Carbs: 2.1 g.
- Fat: 9.2 g.
- Protein: 2.2 g.
- Fiber: 0.9 g.
- Sugar: 0.9 g.

INGREDIENTS:

- 1 cup raw cashews (unsalted)
- ½ cup macadamia nuts (unsalted)
- ½ cup pine nuts
- ½ cup water
- ½ tbsp. coconut oil
- ½ tsp. light miso paste
- 2 tbsp. agar-agar
- 1 tsp. fresh lime juice
- 1 tsp. Himalayan salt

Total number of ingredients: 9

METHOD:

1. Cover the cashews with water in a small bowl and let sit for 4 to 6 hours. Rinse and drain the cashews after soaking. Make sure no water is left.

2. Mix the agar-agar with the ½ cup of water in a small saucepan. Put the pan over medium heat.

3. Bring the agar-agar mixture to a boil. After 1 minute, take it off the heat and set the mixture aside to cool down.

4. Put all the other ingredients—except the coconut oil—in a blender or food processor. Blend until everything is well combined.

5. Add the agar-agar with water and blend again until all ingredients have been fully incorporated.

6. Grease a medium-sized bowl with the coconut oil to prevent the cheese from sticking to the edges. Gently transfer the cheese mixture into the bowl by using a spatula.

7. Refrigerate the bowl, uncovered, for about 3 hours until the cheese is firm; then serve and enjoy!

8. Alternatively, store the cheese in an airtight container in the fridge. Consume within 6 days. Store for a maximum of 60 days in the freezer and thaw at room temperature.

CHEESES

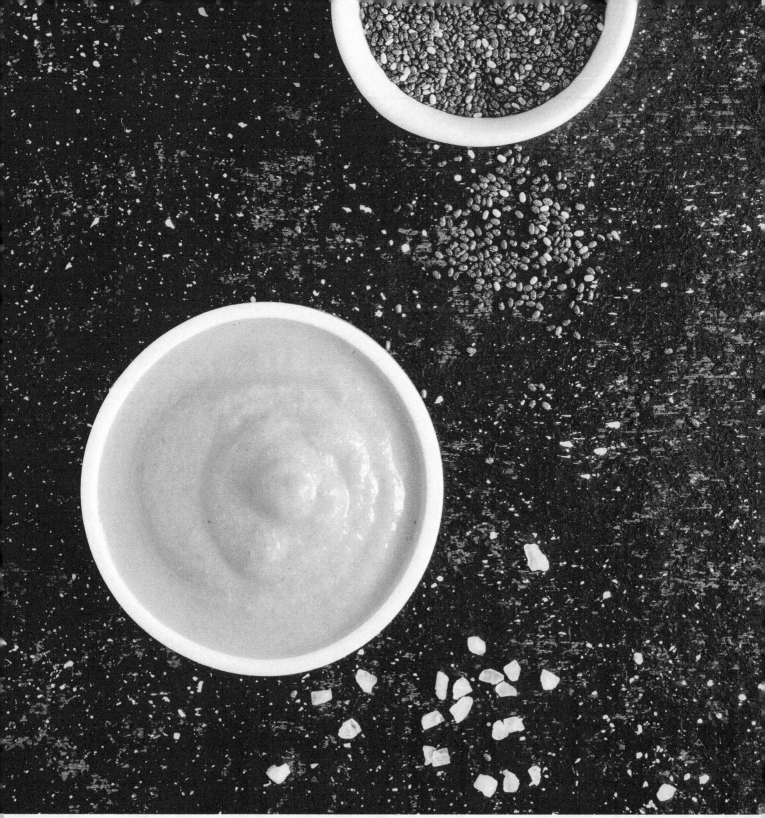

2. Smokey Cheddar Cheese

Serves: 8 / 1 block of cheese | Prep Time: ~20 min |

Nutrition Information
(per serving)
- Calories: 249 kcal
- Net Carbs: 6.9 g.
- Fat: 21.7 g.
- Protein: 6.1 g.
- Fiber: 4.3 g.
- Sugar: 2.6 g.

INGREDIENTS:

- 1 cup raw cashews (unsalted)
- 1 cup macadamia nuts (unsalted)
- 4 tsp. tapioca starch
- 1 cup water
- ¼ cup fresh lime juice
- ¼ cup tahini
- ½ tsp. liquid smoke
- ¼ cup paprika powder
- ½ tsp. ground mustard seeds
- 2 tbsp. onion powder
- 1 tsp. Himalayan salt
- ½ tsp. chili powder
- 1 tbsp. coconut oil

Total number of ingredients: 13

METHOD:

1. Cover the cashews with water in a small bowl and let sit for 4 to 6 hours. Rinse and drain the cashews after soaking. Make sure no water is left.

2. Mix the tapioca starch with the cup of water in a small saucepan. Heat the pan over medium heat.

3. Bring the water with tapioca starch to a boil. After 1 minute, take the pan off the heat and set the mixture aside to cool down.

4. Put all the remaining ingredients—except the coconut oil—in a blender or food processor. Blend until these ingredients are combined into a smooth mixture.

5. Stir in the tapioca starch with water and blend again until all ingredients have fully incorporated.

6. Grease a medium-sized bowl with the coconut oil to prevent the cheese from sticking to the edges. Gently pour the mixture into the bowl.

7. Refrigerate the bowl, uncovered, for about 3 hours until the cheese is firm and ready to enjoy!

8. Alternatively, store the cheese in an airtight container in the fridge and consume within 6 days. Store for a maximum of 60 days in the freezer and thaw at room temperature.

3. Feta Cheese 🌿

Serves: 4 | Prep Time: ~20 min |

Nutrition Information
(per serving)
- Calories: 101 kcal
- Carbs: 5.2 g.
- Net Carbs: 3.8 g.
- Fat: 4.9 g.
- Protein: 10.3 g.
- Fiber:1.4 g.
- Sugar: 0.7 g.

INGREDIENTS:
- 1 13-oz. block extra firm tofu (drained)
- 3 cups water
- ¼ cup apple cider vinegar
- 2 tbsp. dark miso paste
- 1 tsp. ground black pepper
- 2 garlic cloves
- 1 tbsp. sun dried tomatoes (chopped)
- 2 tsp. Himalayan salt

Total number of ingredients: 8

METHOD:
1. Cut the tofu into ½-inch cubes and put them into a medium-sized saucepan with 2 cups of water.

2. Bring the water to a boil over medium-high heat, take the pan off the heat immediately, drain half of the water, and set aside to let it cool down.

3. Pour the vinegar, miso paste, pepper, salt, and the remaining 1 cup of water into a blender or food processor. Blend until everything is well combined.

4. Pour the liquid from the blender into an airtight container. Add the garlic cloves, sundried tomatoes, and the tofu (including the water) to the container.

5. Give the feta cheese a good stir and then store in the fridge or freezer for at least 4 hours before serving.

6. Serve with low-carb crackers, or, enjoy this delicious feta cheese in a healthy salad!

7. Alternatively, store the cheese in an airtight container in the fridge and consume within 6 days. Store for a maximum of 30 days in the freezer and thaw at room temperature.

4. Nut Free Nacho Dip 🌿

Serves: 8 | Prep Time: ~15 min |

Nutrition Information
(per serving)
- Calories: 135 kcal
- Net Carbs: 3.5 g.
- Fat: 12.3 g.
- Protein: 1.8 g.
- Fiber: 5.4 g.
- Sugar: 2.7 g.

INGREDIENTS:
- 1 large eggplant (peeled and cubed)
- 2 medium Hass avocados
  (peeled, pitted, and halved)
- ¼ cup MCT oil
- 2 tsp. nutritional yeast
- 1 jalapeno pepper
- 1 red onion (diced)
- 1 garlic clove (halved)
- ¼ cup fresh cilantro (chopped)
- 1 tbsp. paprika powder
- 1 tsp. cumin seeds
- 1 tsp. dried oregano
- ½ tsp. Himalayan salt

Total number of ingredients: 12

METHOD:
1. Slice the jalapeno in half lengthwise; remove the seeds, stem, and placenta, and discard.
2. Put the jalapeno and all other ingredients in a food processor or blender.
3. Mix everything into a smooth mixture. Use a spatula to scrape down the sides of the blender to make sure everything gets mixed evenly.
4. Transfer the dip to an airtight container.
5. Serve, share, and enjoy!
6. Alternatively, store the cheese in an airtight container in the fridge and consume within 2 days.

Tip: Serve with some celery sticks!

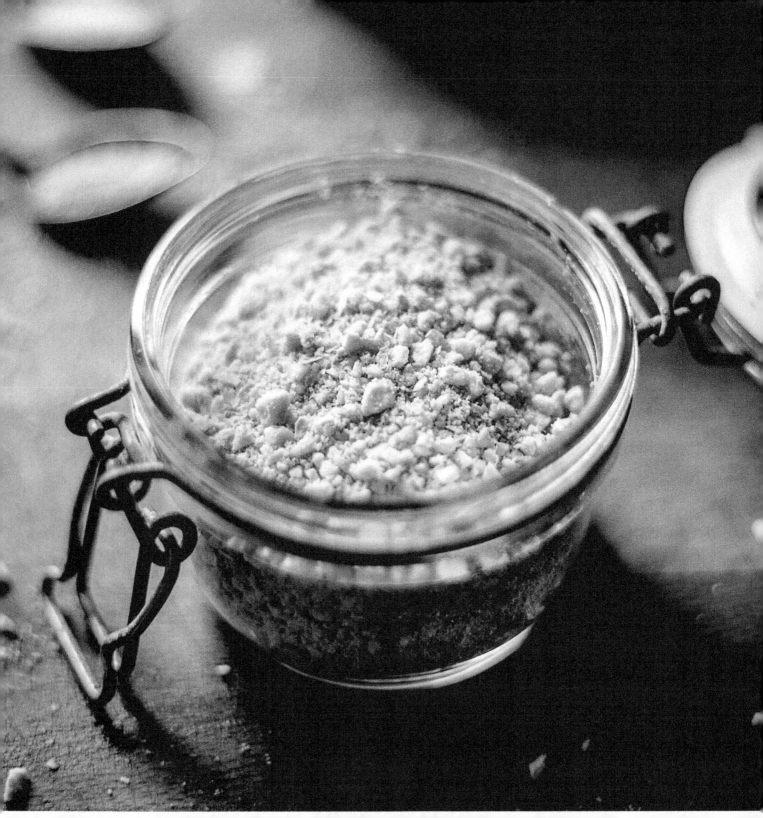

5. Truffle Parmesan Cheese

Serves: 8 | Prep Time: ~30 min |

Nutrition Information
(per serving)
- Calories: 202 kcal
- Net Carbs: 4.4 g.
- Fat: 18.7 g.
- Protein: 4 g.
- Fiber: 1.8 g.
- Sugar: 1.8 g.

INGREDIENTS:
- 1 cup macadamia nuts (unsalted)
- 1 cup raw cashews (unsalted)
- 2 garlic cloves
- ½ tbsp. nutritional yeast
- 2 tbsp. truffle oil
- 1 tsp. agar-agar
- 1 tsp. fresh lime juice
- 1 tsp. dark miso paste

Total number of ingredients: 8

METHOD:

1. Cover the cashews with water in a small bowl and let sit for 4 to 6 hours. Rinse and drain the cashews after soaking. Make sure no water is left.

2. Preheat the oven to 350°F / 175°C, and line a baking sheet with parchment paper.

3. Put the macadamia nuts on a baking sheet and spread them out, so they can roast evenly.

4. Transfer the baking sheet to the oven and roast the macadamia nuts for about 8 minutes, until slightly browned.

5. Take the nuts out of the oven and set them aside, allowing them to cool down.

6. Grease a medium-sized shallow baking dish with ½ tablespoon of truffle oil.

7. Add the soaked cashews, roasted macadamia nuts, and all the remaining ingredients to a blender or food processor. Blend everything into a crumbly mixture.

8. Transfer the crumbly parmesan into the baking dish, spread it out evenly, and firmly press it down until it has fused together into an even layer of cheese.

9. Cover the baking dish with aluminum foil and refrigerate the cheese for 8 hours or until the parmesan is firm.

10. Serve or store the cheese in an airtight container in the fridge and consume within 6 days. Store for a maximum of 60 days in the freezer and thaw at room temperature.

6. Black Olive & Thyme Cheese Spread 🌿

Serves: 16 | Prep Time: ~25 min |

Nutrition Information
(per serving)
- Calories: 118 kcal
- Net Carbs: 0.7 g.
- Fat: 11.9 g.
- Protein: 2 g.
- Fiber: 1.4 g.
- Sugar: 0.7 g.

INGREDIENTS:

- 1 cup macadamia nuts (unsalted)
- 1 cup pine nuts
- 1 tsp. thyme (finely chopped)
- 1 tsp. rosemary (finely chopped)
- 2 tsp. nutritional yeast
- 1 tsp. Himalayan salt
- 10 black olives (pitted, finely chopped)

Total number of ingredients: 7

METHOD:

1. Preheat the oven to 350°F / 175°C, and line a baking sheet with parchment paper.

2. Put the nuts on a baking sheet, and spread them out so they can roast evenly. Transfer the baking sheet to the oven and roast the nuts for about 8 minutes, until slightly browned.

3. Take the nuts out of the oven and set aside for about 4 minutes, allowing them to cool down.

4. Add all ingredients to a blender and process until everything combines into a smooth mixture. Use a spatula to scrape down the sides of the blender container in between blending to make sure everything gets mixed evenly.

5. Serve, share, and enjoy!

6. Alternatively, store the cheese in an airtight container in the fridge and consume within 6 days. Store for a maximum of 60 days in the freezer and thaw at room temperature.

Tip: Serve with some low-carb crackers!

7. Gorgonzola 'Blue' Cheese

Serves: 16 | Prep Time: ~24 hours |

Nutrition Information
(per serving)
- Calories: 101 kcal
- Net Carbs: 2 g.
- Fat: 9.3 g.
- Protein: 2.3 g.
- Fiber: 1 g.
- Sugar: 0.9 g.

INGREDIENTS:

- ½ cup macadamia nuts (unsalted)
- ½ cup pine nuts
- 1 cup raw cashews (unsalted)
- 1 capsule acidophilus
  (probiotic cheese culture)
- ½ tbsp. MCT oil
- ¼ cup unsweetened almond milk
- 1 tsp. ground black pepper
- 1 tsp. Himalayan salt
- 1 tsp. spirulina powder

Total number of ingredients: 9

METHOD:

1. Cover the cashews with water in a small bowl and let sit for 4 to 6 hours. Rinse and drain the cashews after soaking. Make sure no water is left.
2. Preheat the oven to 350°F / 175°C, and line a baking sheet with parchment paper.
3. Spread the macadamia and pine nuts out on the baking sheet so they can roast evenly.
4. Put the baking sheet into the oven and roast the nuts for 8 minutes, until they are slightly browned.
5. Take the nuts out of the oven and allow them to cool down.
6. Grease a 3-inch cheese mold with the MCT oil and set it aside.
7. Add all ingredients—except the spirulina—to the blender or food processor. Blend on medium speed into a smooth mixture. Use a spatula to scrape down the sides of the blender to make sure all the ingredients get incorporated.
8. Transfer the cheese mixture into the greased cheese mold and sprinkle it with the spirulina powder. Use a small teaspoon to create blue marble veins on the cheese, and then cover the mold with parchment paper.
9. Place the cheese into a dehydrator and dehydrate the cheese at 90°F / 32°C for 24 hours.
10. Transfer the dehydrated cheese in the covered mold to the fridge. Allow the cheese to refrigerate for 12 hours.
11. Remove the cheese from the mold to serve in this condition, or, age the cheese in a wine cooler for up to 3 weeks. In case of aging the cheese, rub the outsides of the cheese with fresh sea salt. Refresh the salt every 2 days to prevent any mold. The cheese will develop a blue cheese-like taste, and by aging it, the cheese becomes even more delicious.
12. If the cheese is not aged, store it in airtight container and consume within 6 days.
13. Store the aged cheese in an airtight container and consume within 6 days, or for a maximum of 60 days in the freezer and thaw at room temperature.

8. Smoked Chipotle Cream Cheese 🌿

Serves: 8 | Prep Time: ~20 min |

Nutrition Information
(per serving)
- Calories: 223 kcal
- Net Carbs: 2.9 g.
- Fat: 21.4 g.
- Protein: 4.3 g.
- Fiber: 3.5 g.
- Sugar: 1.9 g.

INGREDIENTS:
- 1 cup macadamia nuts (unsalted)
- ½ cup walnuts
- ½ cup pine nuts
- ¼ cup fresh lemon juice
- 1 tbsp. smoked chipotle pepper
- 1 garlic clove
- 2 tbsp. paprika powder
- ½ tbsp. dried cilantro
- ½ tbsp. dried oregano
- ½ tbsp. dried thyme
- ½ tbsp. dried sweet basil
- 1 tsp. ground cumin

Total number of ingredients: 12

METHOD:
1. Add all ingredients to a blender or food processor. Blend everything into a smooth mixture. Use a spatula to scrape down the sides of the blender to make sure all the ingredients get incorporated.

2. Serve right away and enjoy!

3. Alternatively, store the cheese in an airtight container in the fridge and consume within 6 days. Store for a maximum of 60 days in the freezer and thaw at room temperature.

Tip: Serve with some celery sticks!

9. Classic Cheese Sauce

Serves: 12 | Prep Time: ~20 min |

Nutrition Information
(per serving)
- Calories: 183 kcal
- Carbs: 5.6 g.
- Net Carbs: 2.3 g.
- Fat: 16.8 g.
- Protein: 5.2 g.
- Fiber: 3.4 g.
- Sugar: 2.2 g.

INGREDIENTS:
- 1 cup almonds
- 1 cup macadamia nuts (unsalted)
- 1 tbsp. white wine vinegar
- ½ cup sunflower seed butter
- 2 cups water
- ¼ cup fresh parsley (chopped)
- ¼ cup fresh lovage (chopped)
- 1 tsp. Himalayan salt
- 1 tbsp. nutritional yeast
- 1 tbsp. white truffle oil

Total number of ingredients: 10

METHOD:

1. Cover the almonds and macadamia nuts with water in 2 separate small bowls. Soak the almonds for 12 hours, and the macadamia nuts for 4 to 6 hours. Rinse and drain the nuts after soaking. Make sure no water is left.

2. Transfer the 2 cups of water to a medium-sized saucepan and put it over medium heat. Bring the water to a boil and then add it to a blender or food processor.

3. Add the soaked nuts and the other remaining ingredients to the blender. Blend until everything is combined into a smooth mixture. Use a spatula to scrape down the sides of the blender to make sure all ingredients get incorporated.

4. Serve right away and enjoy!

5. Alternatively, store the cheese in an airtight container in the fridge and consume within 4 days. Store for a maximum of 30 days in the freezer and thaw at room temperature.

Tip: Serve with some low-carb crackers or celery sticks!

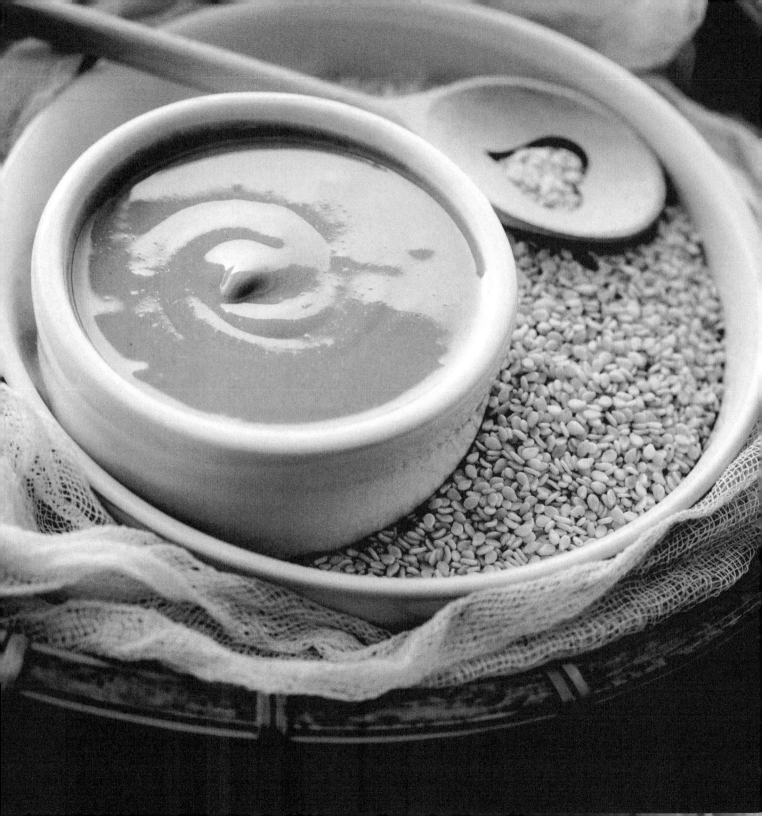

10. Sesame Cheese Spread 🌿

Serves: 8 | Prep Time: ~20 min |

Nutrition Information
(per serving)
- Calories: 111 kcal
- Carbs: 6 g.
- Net Carbs: 3.4 g.
- Fat: 9 g.
- Protein: 3.7 g.
- Fiber: 2.7 g.
- Sugar: 1 g.

INGREDIENTS:
- 1 cup sesame seeds
- 3 tbsp. lemon juice
- 1 tsp. Himalayan salt
- ½ tsp. rice syrup
- 1 tsp. ground black pepper
- ¼ cup fresh lovage (chopped)
- ¼ cup fresh mint (chopped)

Total number of ingredients: 7

METHOD:

1. Cover the sesame seeds in a small bowl filled with water and add 1 tablespoon of lemon juice. Soak the sesame seeds for 12 hours. Rinse and drain the seeds after soaking. Make sure no water is left.

2. Add all the ingredients to a blender or food processor. Blend everything into a smooth mixture. Use a spatula to scrape down the sides of the blender to make sure all the ingredients get incorporated.

3. Serve right away, as a dip for veggies or with some low carb bread, and enjoy!

4. Alternatively, store the cheese in an airtight container in the fridge and consume within 4 days. Store for a maximum of 30 days in the freezer and thaw at room temperature.

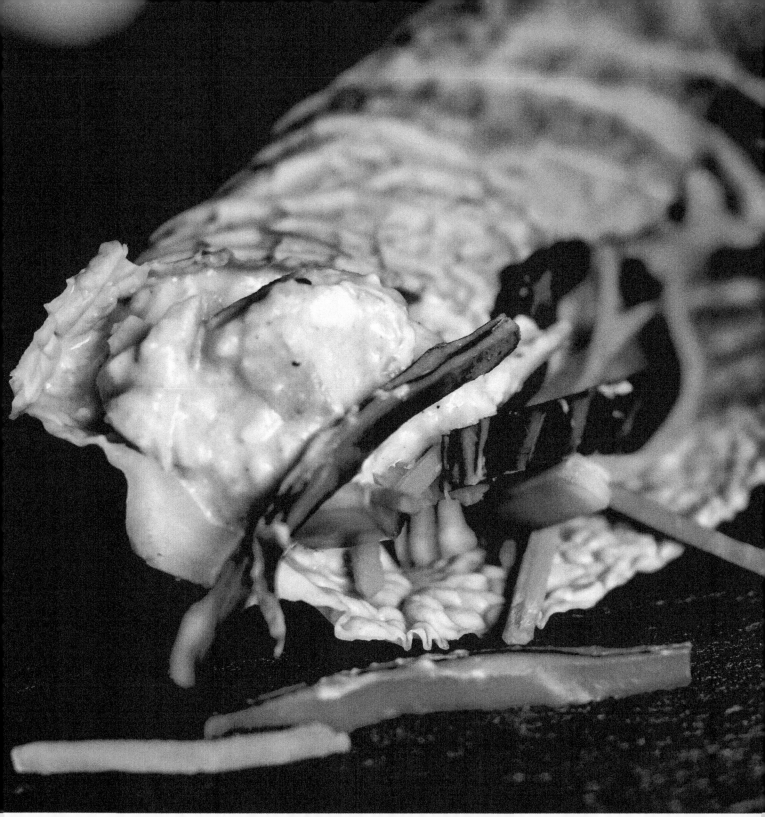

1. Collard Green Wraps with Egg Salad

Nutrition Information
(per serving)
- Calories: 408 kcal
- Net Carbs: 8.8 g.
- Fat: 31.1 g.
- Protein: 22.7 g.
- Fiber: 4.4 g.
- Sugar: 5.7 g.

INGREDIENTS:

Egg Salad:
- 6 large organic eggs (boiled and peeled)
- 7 tbsp. full-fat Greek yogurt
- 1 medium green onion (diced)
- 1 celery stalk (diced)
- 1 tsp. curry powder
- 2 tbsp. avocado oil
- Salt and pepper to taste

Wraps:
- 4 large collard green leaves (rinsed and dried)
- 1 cup carrots (grated)
- ½ cup red cabbage (shredded)
- ½ cup green bell pepper (seeded and sliced)

Total number of ingredients: 12

METHOD:

1. Take a medium-sized bowl, put in the eggs, and crush them into a pulp by using a potato masher or fork.

2. Stir in the yogurt, onion, celery, curry, and avocado oil. Add salt and pepper to taste.

3. Refrigerate the bowl, covered, for 30 minutes.

4. Trim the collard green leaves with a knife. This will help the leaves to serve as wraps.

5. Divide the egg salad over the four leaves. Top each leaf with the grated carrot, shredded cabbage, and bell pepper slices before closing the leaf or rolling it into a wrap.

6. Serve two per person and enjoy!

7. Alternatively, store the egg salad and collard green leaves in the fridge, separated and using airtight containers, and consume within 3 days.

Note: Make sure that the collard green leaves are dry before storing in the fridge; this will prevent early spoilage and soggy leaves.

Tip: Use less egg salad per wrap to make a perfect wrap. Serve the rest on the side and as a separate dish. Add spices like ginger, cumin, or basil for another flavor!

DINNERS

2. Cauliflower & Cheese Pizza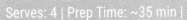

Nutrition Information
(per serving)
- Calories: 318 kcal
- Net Carbs: 9.1 g.
- Fat: 21.1 g.
- Protein: 22.2 g.
- Fiber: 4.2 g.
- Sugar: 5 g.

INGREDIENTS:
- 6 cups cauliflower florets
  (or 15-oz. pack cauliflower rice)
- 2 cups parmesan cheese (grated)
- 1 tsp. onion powder
- ½ tsp. garlic powder
- 2 large organic eggs
- 3 tbsp. tomato paste (unsweetened)
- Handful fresh oregano
- 2 tbsp. olive oil
- Sea salt and ground black pepper to taste

Total number of ingredients: 10

METHOD:
1. Preheat the oven to 400°F / 200°C and line a pizza pan with parchment paper. Grease the paper with 1 tablespoon of olive oil.

2. Put the cauliflower florets in a blender. Pulse the florets into a rice-like substance. Skip this step when using readymade cauliflower rice.

3. Place a medium-sized skillet over medium-high heat and add the cauliflower rice. Heat the rice for about 10 minutes, or until most of the moisture has evaporated.

4. Add the parmesan cheese and seasonings and stir. Then carefully blend in the eggs.

5. Stir the ingredients thoroughly and remove the skillet from the heat.

6. Transfer the dough to a pizza pan. Spread it out and flatten the mixture using a flat wooden spatula.

7. Bake the crust in the oven for 20 minutes.

8. Top the crust with the tomato paste and the remaining ingredients—except the olive oil, salt, and pepper—and bake the pizza for another 5 minutes.

9. Take the pizza out of the oven and cut it into slices. Serve each slice with some olive oil, salt, and pepper to taste on top and enjoy!

10. Alternatively, store the pizza slices in the fridge, using an airtight container and consume within 2 days. Store in the freezer for a maximum of 30 days and thaw at room temperature. Use a microwave or toaster oven to reheat the pizza slices.

Tip: Use more ingredients like cherry tomatoes and more grated parmesan. The oregano can be substituted with fresh rocket.

3. Flaxseed Wraps with Avocado

Serves: 4 | Prep Time: ~25 min |

Nutrition Information
(per serving)
- Calories: 361 kcal
- Net Carbs: 4.8 g.
- Fat: 33.8 g.
- Protein: 7 g.
- Fiber: 15.7 g.
- Sugar: 3.9 g.

INGREDIENTS:

Flaxseed Wraps:
- 1 cup golden flaxseeds
  (or 1 cup ground flaxseed)
- 1 cup water
- Pinch of salt
- ¼ tsp. turmeric
- ¼ tsp. ground ginger
- ¼ tsp. onion powder
- ¼ tsp. garlic powder
- ¼ tsp. paprika

Toppings:
- ¼ cup of full-fat Greek yogurt
  (use coconut yogurt for a vegan dish)
- 4 medium Hass avocados
  (peeled, pitted, and sliced)
- ½ cucumber (peeled and sliced)
- ½ cup cherry tomatoes (halved)
- 2 tbsp. lemon juice
- 2 tbsp. avocado oil
- Salt and black pepper to taste
- Optional: handful fresh mint leaves
- Optional: 2 tbsp. mustard

Total number of ingredients: 18

METHOD:

1. Add the flaxseeds (or ground flaxseed) to a blender. Blend into a very fine meal in order to have it absorb the water.

2. Bring the cup of water to a boil in a small pan.

3. Remove the pan from the heat and mix most of the flaxseed meal with the boiled water using a wooden spoon. Add the remaining spices and salt for the wraps and stir until a dough-like substance is formed.

4. Transfer the dough to a piece of parchment paper covered with a thin layer of the leftover flaxseed meal.

5. Divide the dough into 4 balls. Cover each ball with the surrounding flaxseed meal and then flatten the balls between 2 pieces of parchment paper using a roller pin. Reuse the 2 papers for each wrap, and remove it after flattening.

6. Heat a nonstick medium-sized skillet over medium heat. Cook each wrap for up to 2 minutes, or until the wrap is getting dry. Flip it over and cook it for another minute. Repeat this process for every wrap.

7. Transfer the wraps to a plate and allow them to cool down.

8. Prepare all topping ingredients. Use the yogurt of choice as a base, and put the other topping ingredients on top. If desired, finish with the optional mint leaves and mustard.

9. Carefully fold the wraps up, serve, and enjoy!

10. Alternatively, store the wraps and toppings (separated) in the fridge, using airtight containers and consume within 2 days. The wraps can be frozen for up to 30 days; thaw them at room temperature.

Tip: Add more dry herbs of choice. Supplementing the Greek yogurt with any type of low-carb cheese will guarantee a different flavor!

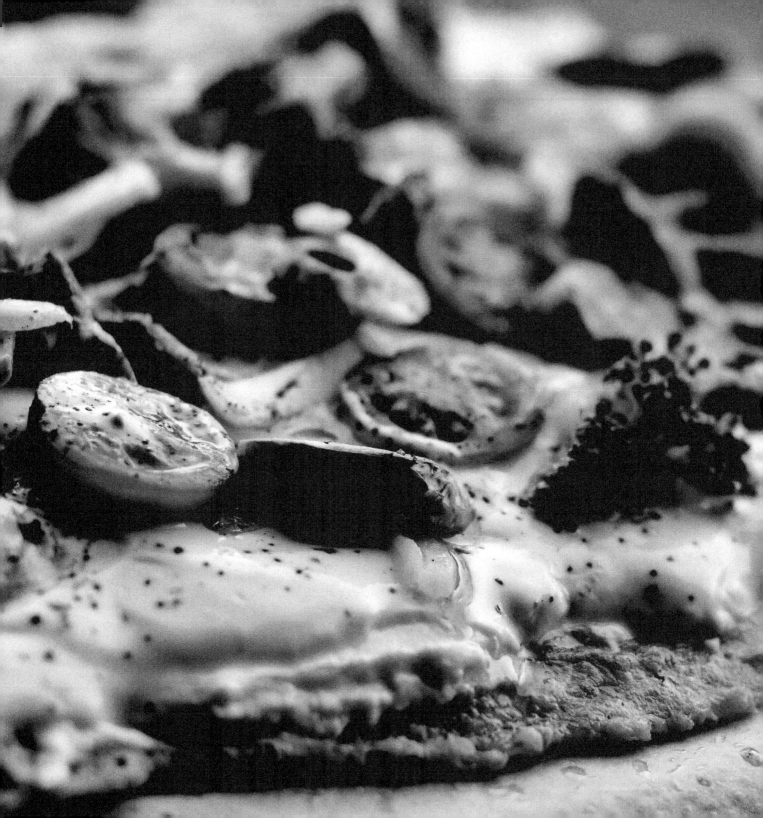

4. Veggie Pizza 🥛 🥚

Serves: 8 | Prep Time: ~35 min |

Nutrition Information
(per serving)
- Calories: 425 kcal
- Net Carbs: 4.3 g.
- Fat: 38.6 g.
- Protein: 14.8 g.
- Fiber: 1.7 g.
- Sugar: 1.9 g.

INGREDIENTS:

Base:
- 2 cups mozzarella cheese (shredded)
- ¾ cup almond flour
- 1 tsp. garlic powder
- 1 large organic egg
- 1 tbsp. olive oil

Topping:
- 2 8-oz. packages cream cheese
- 1 cup full-fat Greek yogurt
- ½ cup broccoli florets (chopped)
- ½ cup cherry tomatoes (halved)
- ½ cup mushrooms (diced)
- ¼ cup green onions (chopped)
- 2 tbsp. olive oil
- Sea salt and ground black pepper to taste

Total number of ingredients: 13

METHOD:

1. Preheat the oven to 425°F / 220°C, and line a baking dish with parchment paper. Coat the paper with 1 tablespoon of olive oil.

2. Melt the mozzarella in a medium-sized bowl by heating it in the microwave on medium for up to 90 seconds.

3. Add the almond flour and garlic powder to the bowl.

4. Stir well using a spoon and then blend in the egg. Reheat the mixture again in the microwave for 20 seconds, if necessary. (The dough needs to be warm in order to be spreadable).

5. Transfer the dough to the baking dish and spread it out into a square-shaped pizza crust.

6. Put the baking dish in the oven and bake the pizza crust for 10 minutes, until lightly brown.

7. Take the crust out of the oven and top it with all the topping ingredients—except the olive oil, salt, and pepper.

8. Turn the oven heat down to 300°F / 150°C and reheat the pizza for 5 minutes before serving.

9. Slice the pizza into 8 servings. Top each slice with some olive oil, salt, and pepper to taste.

10. Serve right away, or alternatively, store the pizza slices in the fridge in an airtight container and consume within 2 days. Store in the freezer for a maximum of 30 days and thaw at room temperature. Use a microwave or toaster oven to reheat the pizza slices.

Tip: Add more mozzarella and fresh vegetables—like diced bell peppers and red onions—on top of the pizza. Spices like chili flakes will also contribute to the flavor.

5. Scrambled Fried Tofu with Cheese

Nutrition Information
(per serving)
- Calories: 447 kcal
- Net Carbs: 8.3 g.
- Fat: 33 g.
- Protein: 28.7 g.
- Fiber: 4.5 g.
- Sugar: 3.5 g.

INGREDIENTS:
- 2 8-oz. packages firm tofu (drained)
- ½ cup cheddar cheese (shredded)
- 2 tbsp. olive oil
- 1 green bell pepper (seeded and diced)
- 2 scallions (chopped)
- 1 tsp. garlic powder
- 1 tsp. onion powder
- ½ tsp. turmeric
- Sea salt and black pepper to taste
- Optional: 1 medium tomato (diced)

Total number of ingredients: 11

METHOD:

1. Cut the tofu into tiny cubes and drain any liquid that is left.

2. Take a large skillet and heat it over medium-high heat. Add the olive oil and tofu cubes. Crush the tofu into tiny crumbles by using a wooden spatula while stirring.

3. Add the diced bell pepper and chopped scallions. Stir continuously until the tofu starts to brown.

4. Blend in the spices and heat the ingredients for another 8 minutes. Finally, add the cheese and, if desired, the optional diced tomato.

5. Stir the ingredients for another minute, and then take the skillet off the heat. Drain any excess liquid from the tofu cheese scramble.

6. Top the dish with more salt and pepper to taste before serving.

7. Alternatively, store the tofu cheese scramble in an airtight container in the fridge, and consume within 4 days. Store in the freezer for a maximum of 30 days and thaw at room temperature. Use a microwave, toaster oven, or pan to reheat the tofu cheese scramble.

Tip: Serve this mixture with the Protein Nut 'N Seed Bread (page 41).

6. Cheddar Tofu

Serves: 2 | Prep Time: ~30 min |

Nutrition Information
(per serving)
- Calories: 513 kcal
- Net Carbs: 4.5 g.
- Fat: 45.4 g.
- Protein: 21.7 g.
- Fiber: 1.1 g.
- Sugar: 0.3 g.

INGREDIENTS:
- 1 cup coconut milk
- 1 cup cheddar cheese (shredded)
- 1 cup firm tofu (drained)
- ½ tsp. sea salt
- 1 tsp. gellan gum

Total number of ingredients: 5

METHOD:

1. Heat up a baking tray in the oven at 200°F / 100°C.

2. Put a medium-sized pot over medium heat and add the coconut milk and cheese.

3. Allow the mixture to cook for 5 minutes while constantly stirring. Then turn off the heat, cover the pot, and allow the mixture to sit for 20 minutes.

4. Filter the milk through a sieve and set the solid cheese aside which can be served as a snack or side dish later.

5. Put the cheddar milk, tofu, and salt in a blender. Blend the ingredients into a silky-smooth mixture.

6. Pour the mixture into the previously used pot and stir in the gellan gum.

7. Reheat the pot over medium heat until the mixture almost reaches a boiling point. This is necessary to get the gellan gum fully hydrated.

8. Stir and pour the mixture into the warmed baking dish. Try to do so as quickly as possible, as the gellan gum sets when it cools down.

9. Allow the mixture to harden up as it cools down. Slice it up, serve and enjoy!

10. Alternatively, store the cheddar tofu in the fridge, using an airtight container, and consume within 4 days. Store in the freezer for a maximum of 30 days and thaw at room temperature. Use a microwave or toaster oven to reheat the cheddar tofu.

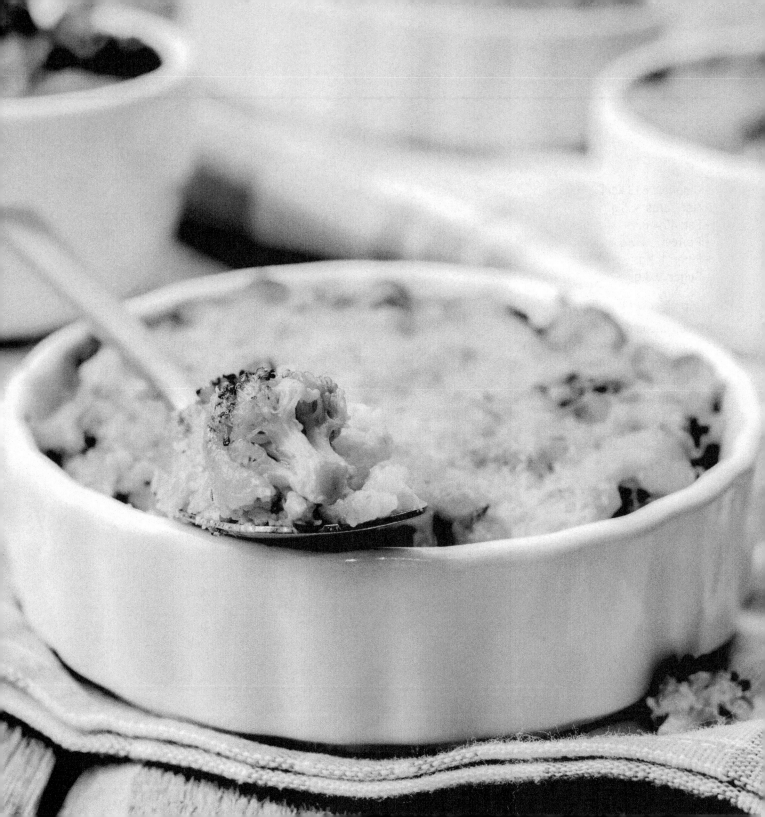

7. Cheesy Broccoli Casserole 🥛 🥚

Serves: 3 | Prep Time: ~30 min |

Nutrition Information
(per serving)
- Calories: 633 kcal
- Net Carbs: 5.1 g.
- Fat: 60.1 g.
- Protein: 17.6 g.
- Fiber: 1.8 g.
- Sugar: 1.5 g.

INGREDIENTS:

- 3 cups broccoli florets (diced)
- 2 tbsp. warm water
- 1 cup cream cheese
- 1 cup cheddar cheese (grated)
- ¼ cup full-fat mayonnaise
- 1 tbsp. avocado oil
- 1 tsp. garlic powder
- ½ tsp. ground black pepper
- Pinch of salt

Total number of ingredients: 9

METHOD:

1. Preheat the oven to 350°F / 175°C.
2. Add the diced broccoli and water to a casserole dish.
3. Add the cheese, mayonnaise, avocado oil, and spices, and stir until all the ingredients are well combined.
4. Top the dish with some additional ground black pepper and salt to taste.
5. Transfer the casserole dish into the oven. Bake the casserole for about 10 minutes, until the crust starts to brown.
6. Allow the casserole to cool down, serve, and enjoy!
7. Alternatively, store the broccoli casserole in an airtight container in the fridge, and consume within 4 days. Store in the freezer for a maximum of 30 days and thaw at room temperature. Use a microwave, toaster oven, or pan to reheat the broccoli casserole.

Tip: Top the dish with more cheddar or grated parmesan. Include white pepper for another flavor!

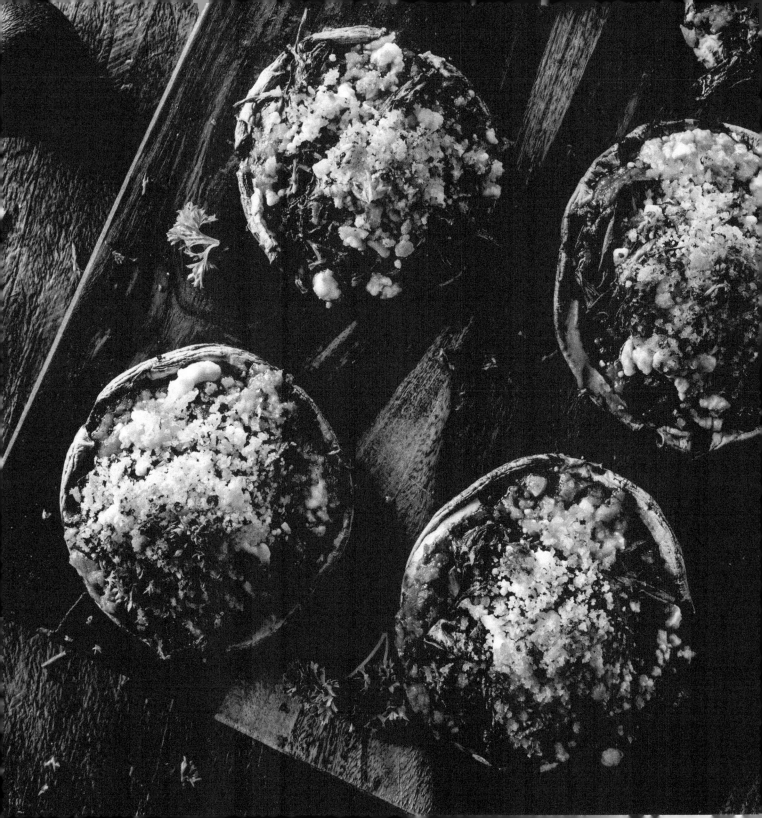

8. Stuffed Green Portobello Caps

Serves: 4 | Prep Time: ~25 min |

Nutrition Information
(per serving)
- Calories: 279 kcal
- Net Carbs: 5.7 g.
- Fat: 23.3 g.
- Protein: 11.4 g.
- Fiber: 3.1 g.
- Sugar: 2.8 g.

INGREDIENTS:
- 4 portobello mushroom caps (stemless)
- 4 tbsp. grass-fed butter
- 1 cup frozen spinach (defrosted and drained)
- 1 cup artichoke hearts (drained and chopped)
- ½ cup parmesan cheese (grated)
- ¼ cup cream cheese
- ½ cup mozzarella cheese
- ½ tbsp. garlic powder
- Sea salt and black pepper to taste

Total number of ingredients: 10

METHOD:
1. Preheat the oven to 375°F / 190°C, and line a baking tray with aluminum foil.
2. Choose to leave the innards of the mushrooms in or take them out. Cover each cap with the grass-fed butter on both sides. Use warm butter to make this step easier.
3. Place the caps on the baking tray and transfer the tray to the oven. Broil the caps for 5 minutes, then flip them over and broil for another 5 minutes.
4. Get rid of any excess water left in the spinach using a sieve and paper towels.
5. Mix the spinach, artichoke, parmesan cheese, cream cheese, garlic powder, salt, and pepper in a medium-sized bowl.
6. Top each mushroom cap with this mixture and distribute it evenly.
7. Finally, add the mozzarella and bake the caps for another 10-12 minutes, until all cheese has melted. Top the stuffed cap with some additional salt and pepper to taste.
8. Take the tray out of the oven, allow the caps to cool down before serving, and enjoy!
9. Alternatively, store the stuffed portobello caps in an airtight container in the fridge, and consume within 3 days. Store in the freezer for a maximum of 30 days and thaw at room temperature. Use a microwave or toaster oven to reheat the stuffed portobello caps.

Tip: Add sour cream and more butter to the stuffing. Top the caps with cayenne pepper or chili flakes for a spicy bite!

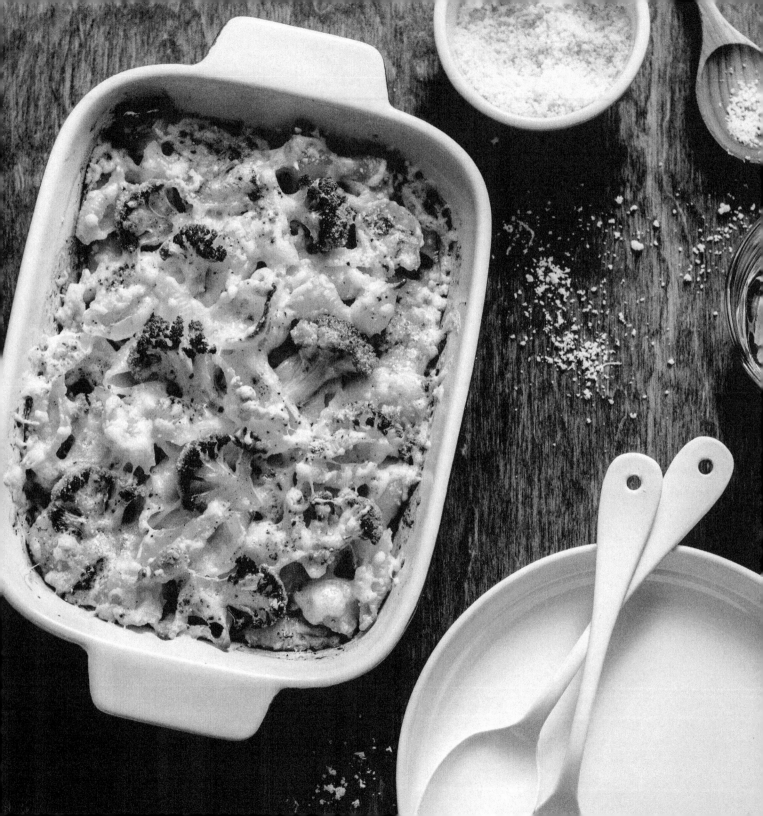

9. Keto Mac 'N Cheese

Nutrition Information
(per serving)
- Calories: 572 kcal
- Net Carbs: 7.6 g.
- Fat: 53.1 g.
- Protein: 15.3 g.
- Fiber: 3.2 g.
- Sugar: 3.2 g.

INGREDIENTS:
- 1 large cauliflower (stems removed)
- 1 cup heavy cream
- ½ cup cheddar cheese (shredded)
- ½ cup fontina cheese (shredded)
- ¼ cup cream cheese
- 1 tbsp. olive oil
- 2 tsp. paprika powder
- 1 tsp. cayenne pepper
- Sea salt and black pepper to taste

Total number of ingredients: 10

METHOD:

1. Preheat the oven to 375°F / 190°C, and coat a deep baking tray with the olive oil.
2. Cut the cauliflower into tiny florets.
3. Fill a medium-sized pot with water and bring to a boil over medium heat.
4. Steam the cauliflower chunks in a sieve above the pot for 5 minutes.
5. Turn the heat down to low, take off the pot, and get rid of the water. Set the cauliflower aside for now.
6. Put the pot back on the stove and add the heavy cream, cheeses, and spices.
7. Turn the heat back up to medium and stir the ingredients until everything is mixed together.
8. Add the cauliflower chunks and cover the pot.
9. Carefully shake the pot to toss and coat the steamed cauliflower chunks.
10. Transfer the mixture into the greased baking dish and bake the mac 'n cheese in the oven for 25-30 minutes, until the top layer is golden brown.
11. Take the dish out of the oven and cover it with some additional salt and pepper to taste.
12. Allow the dish to cool down before serving and enjoy!
13. Alternatively, store the mac 'n cheese in the fridge in an airtight container, and consume within 3 days. Store in the freezer for a maximum of 30 days and thaw at room temperature. Use a microwave or toaster oven to reheat the mac 'n cheese.

Tip: Incorporate scrambled tofu or tempeh for more protein.

10. Portobello Pizzas

Serves: 4 | Prep Time: ~35 min |

Nutrition Information
(per serving)
- Calories: 303 kcal
- Net Carbs: 4.4 g.
- Fat: 26.7 g.
- Protein: 11 g.
- Fiber: 2.3 g.
- Sugar: 3.3 g.

INGREDIENTS:
- 4 portobello mushroom caps (stemless)
- 1 8-oz. package firm tofu (drained)
- 1 medium tomato (sliced)
- ½ cup mozzarella cheese (shredded; alternatively use cheddar)
- ½ cup fresh spinach
- 6 tbsp. olive oil
- ½ tsp. garlic powder
- Sea salt and black pepper to taste
- Optional: ¼ cup fresh basil

Total number of ingredients: 10

METHOD:

1. Preheat the oven to 300°F / 150°C, and line a baking tray with parchment paper.

2. Cut the tofu into 4 equal slices and set aside.

3. Choose to leave the innards of the mushroom in or take them out. Divide 1 tablespoon of olive oil per portobello cap, either on top of the innards or inside the trimmed portobello caps.

4. Top the caps with the garlic powder and a pinch of salt and pepper.

5. Transfer the caps to the baking tray and put in the oven. Broil the caps for 5 minutes. Flip over the caps and divide the final 2 tablespoons of olive oil over the top sides of the portobello caps. Broil the top side in the oven for another 3 minutes.

6. Take out the tray, flip the caps back over with the bottom facing up, and top each cap with the spinach leaves, tomato slices, tofu slices, and mozzarella cheese. The cheese should be on top. Add more salt and pepper to taste if desired.

7. Transfer the baking tray back to the oven and broil the portobello pizzas for 2 minutes.

8. Finally add the optional fresh basil, if desired, and more salt and pepper to taste.

9. Broil the pizzas for another 2 minutes. Make sure the mozzarella cheese melts.

10. Take the tray out, allow the portobello pizzas to cool down for a minute before serving, and enjoy!

11. Alternatively, store the portobello pizzas in the fridge, using an airtight container, and consume within 4 days. Store in the freezer for a maximum of 30 days and thaw at room temperature. Use a microwave or toaster oven to reheat the portobello pizzas.

Tip: Incorporate cheese, like parmesan or cheddar. Switch the fresh spinach and basil leaves for a layer of pesto.

11. Eggplant & Cheese Casserole

Nutrition Information
(per serving)
- Calories: 496 kcal
- Net Carbs: 8.1 g.
- Fat: 38.8 g.
- Protein: 28 g.
- Fiber: 4.2 g.
- Sugar: 4.6 g.

INGREDIENTS:

- 2 medium eggplants
  (with or without skin)
- 2 tbsp. olive oil
- 1½ cups mozzarella cheese (grated)
- 1½ cups simple marinara sauce
  (page 35)
- ½ cup parmesan cheese
- Sea salt to taste
- 1 medium tomato (sliced)
- Optional: black pepper to taste
- Optional: handful fresh basil (chopped)

Total number of ingredients: 9

METHOD:

1. Preheat the oven to 350°F / 175°C, and line a baking tray with aluminum foil. Grease the foil with 1 tablespoon of olive oil.

2. Slice the eggplant into thin slices, and dry these with paper towels to get rid of any water. Sprinkle some salt on top of the slices and transfer them to the greased baking tray.

3. Bake the slices for 3 minutes in the oven, then flip them over. Cook for another 3 minutes.

4. Take the tray out of the oven and set the slices aside. Do not turn off the oven.

5. Take a casserole dish and grease it with the remaining table-spoon of olive oil.

6. Add ⅓ of the simple marinara sauce, then add parmesan cheese, a layer of broiled eggplant slices, and then mozzarella.

7. Repeat this until these ingredients—except some remaining parmesan cheese—are all incorporated in the dish.

8. Top the eggplant & cheese with a layer of sliced tomatoes, followed with the final layer of parmesan cheese and optional black pepper.

9. Bake the dish in the oven up to 20 minutes, or until the top layer of cheese is golden brown.

10. Take the casserole out of the oven and allow the dish to cool before topping it with the optional basil, if desired. Slice, serve, and enjoy!

11. Alternatively, store the eggplant casserole in an airtight container in the fridge, and consume within 3 days. Store in the freezer for a maximum of 30 days, and thaw at room temperature. Use a microwave or toaster oven to reheat the eggplant casserole.

Tip: Use more or less cheese to your liking. Add as much basil and oregano as your taste buds can handle!

12. Green Curry Tofu with Cauliflower Rice

Serves: 4 | Prep Time: ~30 min |

Nutrition Information
(per serving)
- Calories: 177 kcal
- Net. Carbs: 7.9 g.
- Fat: 13.5 g.
- Protein: 6 g.
- Fiber: 3.6 g.
- Sugar: 2.8 g.

INGREDIENTS:
- 4 oz. silken tofu (drained)
- 1 tbsp. extra virgin coconut oil
- ½ cup coconut cream
- 1½ cups cauliflower rice
  (or blend 3-4 cups stemless
  cauliflower florets)
- 1 stalk lemongrass (sliced)
- ½ cup green peas
- ½ cup fresh basil
- ½ cup fresh cilantro
- 4 tbsp. soy sauce
- 3 garlic cloves (minced)
- 4 small green chilis
- 1½ tbsp. ginger
- 2 tbsp. green curry paste
- 1 lime
- 1 tbsp. canola oil
- ½ tsp. ground cumin
- ½ tsp. turmeric
- 1 tsp. salt

Total number of ingredients: 18

METHOD:
1. Preheat the oven to 350°F / 180°C, and line a baking sheet with parchment paper.
2. Cut the tofu into tiny cubes. Add the coconut oil and 1 tablespoon of soy sauce and make sure that all the cubes are greased.
3. Spread out the tofu on the baking sheet and transfer it to the oven. Bake the tofu cubes for 12-15 minutes.
4. Put all the ingredients—except the canola oil, cauliflower rice, remaining soy sauce, green peas, and salt—in a blender. Blend these ingredients into a liquid while adding 2 tablespoons of soy sauce.
5. Take a large skillet and heat it over medium heat. Add the canola oil, green curry paste, green peas, and the blended vegetables.
6. Stir in the coconut cream and let the mixture cook for about 5 minutes while stirring.
7. Add the cauliflower rice and the last tablespoon of soy sauce to the skillet.
8. Cook the mixture for 5 minutes while occasionally stirring.
9. Take the tofu out of the oven and sprinkle it with the salt.
10. Carefully add the tofu cubes to the dish and take the skillet off the heat.
11. Allow the food to cool down for about 10 minutes before serving and enjoy!
12. Alternatively, store the green curry tofu and the cauliflower rice, separated, in the fridge; use airtight containers and consume within 3 days. Store in the freezer for a maximum of 30 days and thaw at room temperature. Use a microwave or toaster oven to reheat green curry tofu with cauliflower rice.

Note: Use less soy sauce and little or no salt for less sodium.

Tip: Add more low-carb (green) vegetables. Broccoli, green bell peppers, onions and green beans are great examples.

13. Veg 'N Cheese Casserole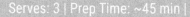

Nutrition Information
(per serving)
- Calories: 359 kcal
- Net Carbs: 6.8 g.
- Fat: 32.7 g.
- Protein: 9 g.
- Fiber: 3.4 g.
- Sugar: 1.8 g.

INGREDIENTS:
- ¼ cup firm tofu (drained)
- 1 tbsp. grass-fed butter
- ½ cup cream cheese
- 1/6 cup full-fat mayonnaise
- 1/6 cup sour cream
- 1 cup spinach (chopped)
- 1¼ cups artichoke hearts (chopped)
- ½ small red onion (diced)
- ½ tsp. dried cayenne pepper
- ¼ tsp. garlic powder
- ¼ cup parmesan cheese (shredded)
- Sea salt and ground black pepper to taste

Total number of ingredients: 13

METHOD:
1. Preheat the oven to 400°F / 200°C.
2. Put a large skillet over medium heat and add the butter and diced onions. Sauté the onions until translucent.
3. Stir in the chopped spinach, artichoke hearts, and cayenne pepper. Add salt and pepper to taste.
4. Take a large bowl and add the cream cheese, mayonnaise, sour cream, and garlic powder. Use a whisk to incorporate these ingredients, and then transfer the mixture to the skillet.
5. Crumble the tofu into small pieces and add these to the skillet.
6. Transfer the content of the skillet to a casserole dish or a pan suitable for the oven.
7. Top the casserole with the parmesan cheese and additional salt and pepper to taste.
8. Bake the casserole for 20 minutes, until the cheese is golden brown.
9. Take the casserole dish out of the oven and allow it to cool for a few minutes before serving. Then enjoy!
10. Alternatively, store the casserole in the fridge in an airtight container, and consume within 3 days. Store in the freezer for a maximum of 30 days and thaw at room temperature. Use a microwave, toaster oven, or pan to reheat the casserole.

Tip: Substitute the fresh spinach with frozen spinach and the artichoke hearts with a canned version for faster preparation.

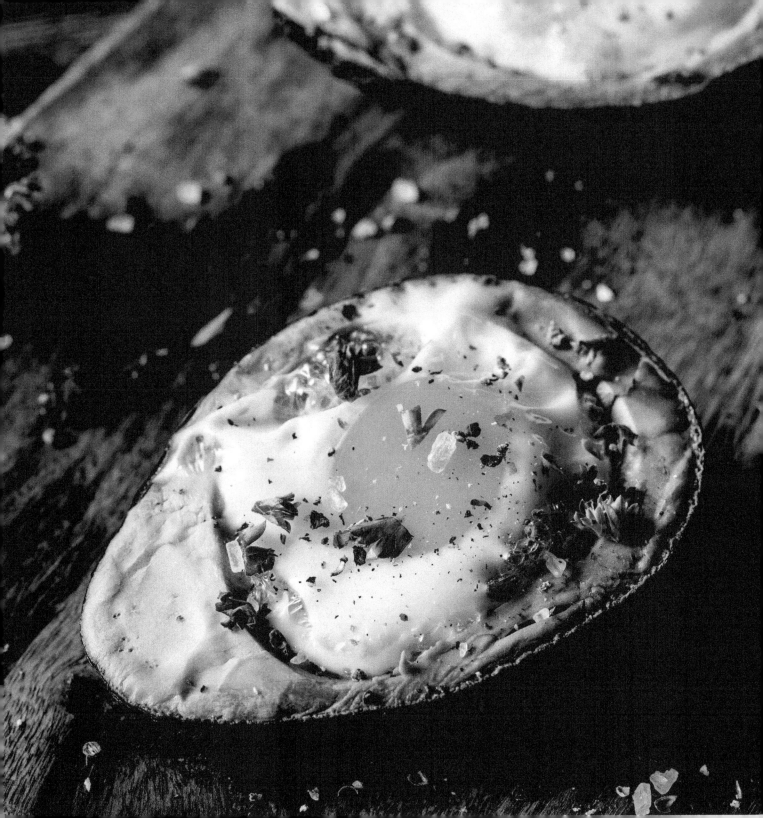

14. Egg-Stuffed Avocados

Serves: 2 | Prep Time: ~30 min |

Nutrition Information
(per serving)
- Calories: 411 kcal
- Net Carbs: 6.8 g.
- Fat: 34.8 g.
- Protein: 15 g.
- Fiber: 13.2 g.
- Sugar: 4 g.

INGREDIENTS:
- 4 medium organic eggs
- 2 large Hass avocados
  (peeled, pitted, and halved)
- ¼ cup fresh parsley (chopped)
- ½ tbsp. smoked chipotle pepper
- 1 tsp. garlic powder
- 1 tsp. ground cumin seeds
- 1 tsp. onion powder
- 1 tsp. dried oregano
- Sea salt to taste
- 1 tbsp. lemon juice
- 1 tbsp. fresh cilantro (chopped)

Total number of ingredients: 11

METHOD:
1. Preheat oven at 425°F / 220°C, and line a baking dish with parchment paper.

2. Put the avocado halves on the baking dish. Position the 4 halves against the edges of the sheet, so they won't tip over.

3. Carefully crack the eggs open, making sure to keep the yolks intact.

4. Use a tablespoon to transfer 1 egg yolk into each hole of the avocado halves.

5. Top the yolks in the avocado halves with the egg white.

6. Season the avocado halves with chipotle pepper, garlic powder, onion powder, ground cumin seeds, oregano, and salt to taste.

7. Carefully transfer the baking dish to the oven and bake the stuffed avocado halves until the eggs are cooked, or for about 12 minutes.

8. Take the baking dish out of the oven and allow the stuffed avocado halves to cool down.

9. Sprinkle the lemon juice on top of the avocado halves, garnish with cilantro, serve, and enjoy!

10. Storing and reheating the egg filled avocadoes is not recommended.

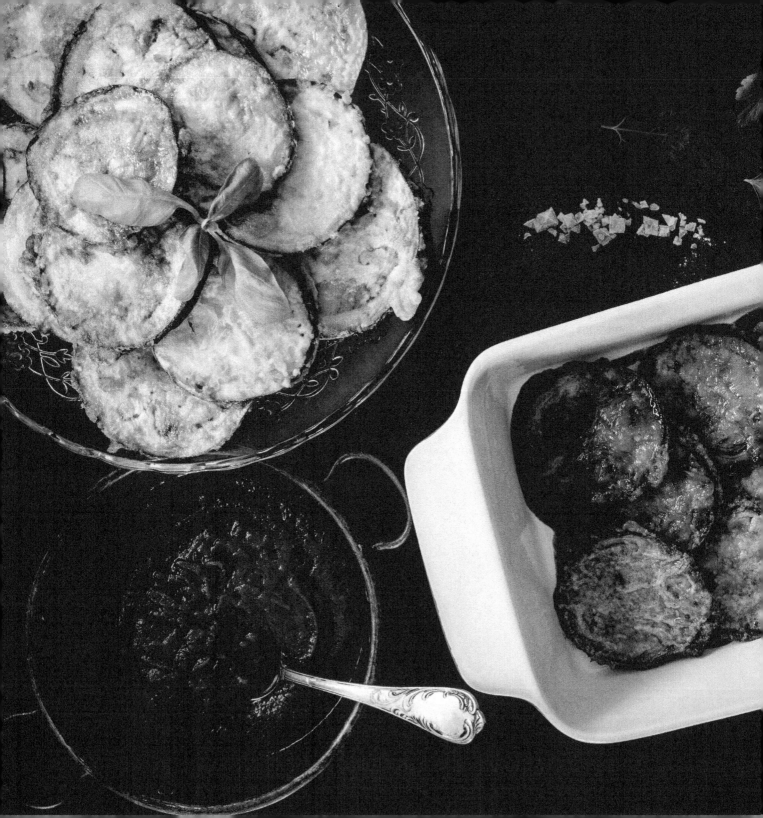

15. Eggplant Parmigiana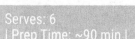

Nutrition Information
(per serving)
- Calories: 466 kcal
- Net Carbs: 12.3 g.
- Fat: 33 g.
- Protein: 29 g.
- Fiber: 8.5 g.
- Sugar: 6.7 g.

INGREDIENTS:
- 3 large eggplants
- 2 tbsp. extra virgin olive oil
- ¼ cup yellow onion (diced)
- 3 medium garlic cloves (minced)
- 1 tbsp. Italian seasoning
- 3 cups simple marinara sauce (page 35)
- 2 cups full-fat Ricotta cheese
- 4 cups mozzarella cheese (shredded)
- ¼ cup fresh basil (chopped)
- 2 tsp. garlic powder
- 1 tbsp. fresh parsley (chopped)
- Kosher salt and ground black pepper to taste

Total number of ingredients: 13

METHOD:
1. Preheat the oven to 375°F / 190°C, and line a baking tray with aluminum foil.
2. Cut the ends off the eggplants and slice them lengthwise into ¼-inch-thick slices.
3. Put the eggplant slices on a dry cutting board and sprinkle with a pinch of salt on both sides. Allow the slices to sit for 30 minutes.
4. Dry the eggplant slices using paper towels.
5. Grease the baking tray with 1 tablespoon of olive oil, and put the dried eggplant slices on it.
6. Broil the slices in the oven for 5 minutes, then flip them over and broil for another 5 minutes. Take the tray out and set it aside. Do not turn off the oven.
7. Place a large skillet over medium-high heat and add the other 1 tablespoon of olive oil.
8. Add the onions, garlic, and Italian seasoning. Top with salt and pepper to taste.
9. Sauté the vegetables for about 5 minutes, until the onions are translucent.
10. Add the simple marinara sauce, stir, and cook the mixture for an additional 5 minutes before removing the pan from the heat.
11. Take a large bowl and mix the ricotta cheese, 1 cup of mozzarella cheese, garlic powder, and basil.
12. Use a large baking dish and spread a small amount of marinara sauce on the bottom of the pan.
13. Start building the lasagna in layers of ingredients, starting with the eggplant, followed by a layer of the ricotta mixture, a layer of mozzarella cheese, and finally another layer of marinara sauce.
14. Continue doing this until the baking dish is filled or all the ingredients—except the mozzarella cheese and parsley—are used. Make sure the last layer is marinara sauce. Set the remaining mozzarella and parsley aside for later.
15. Cover the baking dish with aluminum foil. Turn up the heat of the oven to 400°F / 200°C and bake the parmigiana for 25-30 minutes.
16. Remove the foil and top the dish with the remaining mozzarella cheese. Sprinkle some freshly chopped parsley on top, and put the parmigiana back in the oven for an additional 10-15 minutes, until the cheese melts and the top layer turns golden brown.
17. Remove the baking dish from the oven and allow the parmigiana to cool for 15 minutes.
18. Cut the eggplant parmigiana into the desired number of portions, serve with salt and pepper to taste, and enjoy!
19. Alternatively, store the parmigiana in the fridge, using an airtight container, and consume within 4 days. Store in the freezer for a maximum of 30 days and thaw at room temperature. Use a microwave, toaster oven or pan to reheat the parmigiana.

Tip: Incorporate some tofu, seitan, or eggs in this dish for extra protein. A small amount of breadcrumbs can improve both taste and texture.

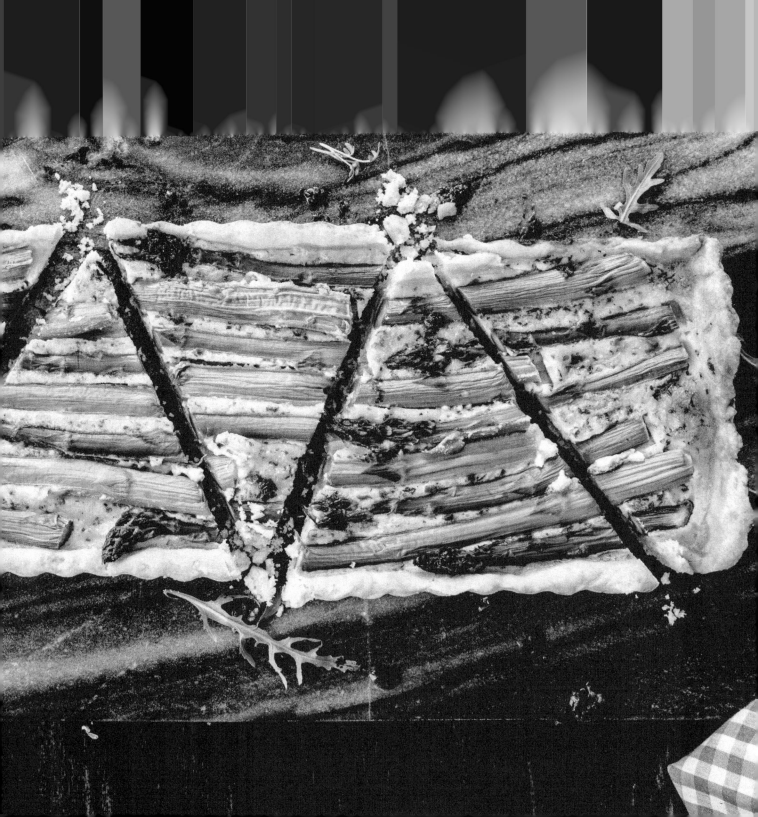

16. Asparagus Quiche

Nutrition Information
(per serving)
- Calories: 315 kcal
- Net Carbs: 4.1 g.
- Fat: 25.3 g.
- Protein: 17.1 g.
- Fiber: 2.4 g.
- Sugar: 2.3 g.

INGREDIENTS:

- 1 cup asparagus (stems removed and chopped)
- 2 cups mozzarella (shredded)
- 2 tbsp. extra virgin coconut oil
- 1½ cups spinach leaves (chopped)
- 2 medium garlic cloves (minced)
- ½ tsp. nutmeg
- 1 green onion (diced)
- 4 large organic eggs
- 2 tbsp. parmesan cheese (grated)
- Sea salt and black pepper to taste
- Optional: 1 tsp. cayenne pepper

Total number of ingredients: 11

METHOD:

1. Preheat the oven to 375°F / 190°C.
2. Heat up a medium-sized skillet over medium heat.
3. Grill the asparagus pieces for up to 2 minutes while occasionally stirring. Take the skillet off the heat and set the asparagus aside.
4. Take a pie pan and grease it with the coconut oil.
5. Combine the eggs with the minced garlic, nutmeg, and most of the mozzarella in a medium-sized bowl. Save ¼ cup of mozzarella cheese and ¼ cup of the egg mixture for the topping.
6. Add the main portion of the egg mixture and the chopped spinach into the greased pie pan.
7. Put a layer of the grilled asparagus and diced green onions on top of the egg and spinach.
8. Add the reserved part of the egg mixture and mozzarella cheese on top.
9. Top the uncooked quiche with salt, black pepper, and the optional cayenne pepper, if desired, to taste.
10. Cover the quiche with the parmesan cheese and transfer it to the oven.
11. Bake the quiche for 25-30 minutes, until the cheese starts to get brown. Allow the quiche to cool down for a few minutes.
12. Slice the quiche into the desired number of portions, serve, and enjoy!
13. Alternatively, store the quiche in an airtight container in the fridge, and consume within 3 days. Store in the freezer for a maximum of 30 days and thaw at room temperature. Use a microwave or toaster oven to reheat the quiche.

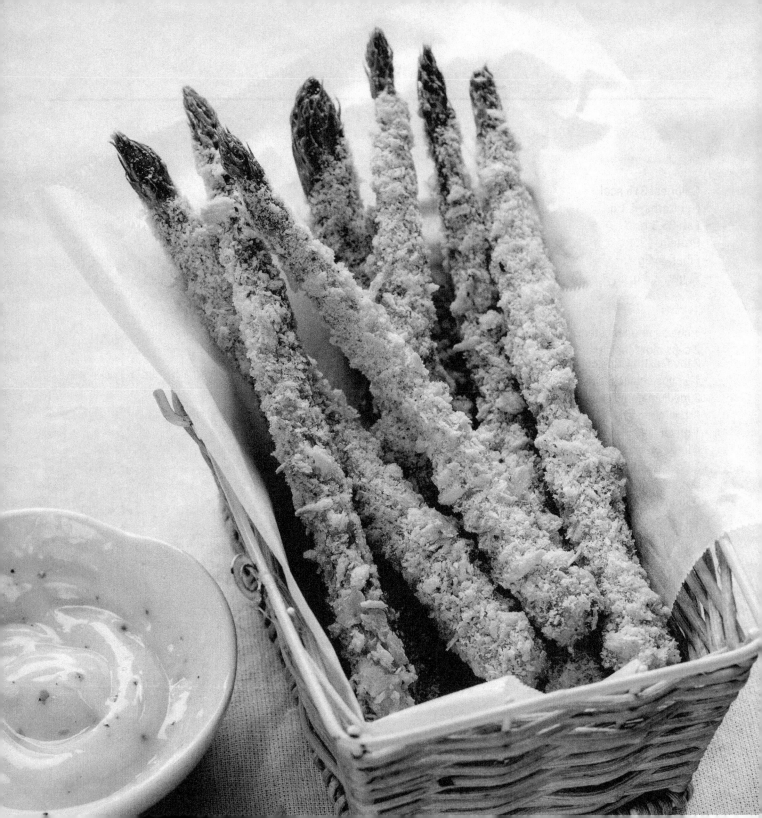

17. Crunchy Fried Asparagus 🍃

Serves: 4 | Prep Time: ~35 min |

Nutrition Information
(per serving)
- Calories: 247 kcal
- Net Carbs: 3.8 g.
- Fat: 22 g.
- Protein: 7.7 g.
- Fiber: 4.2 g.
- Sugar: 1.6 g.

INGREDIENTS:
- 10 asparagus spears
- 1 cup almond flour
- 2 tbsp. olive oil (alternatively use coconut oil)
- 1 tsp. sea salt
- ½ tsp. black pepper
- 1 tsp. smoked paprika
- 2 tsp. low-carb maple syrup
- 1½ tbsp. nutritional yeast

Total number of ingredients: 8

METHOD:

1. Preheat the oven to 400°F / 200°C, and line a baking sheet with parchment paper.

2. Cut the asparagus in half and transfer these halves to a medium-sized bowl.

3. Add the spices to the bowl and stir.

4. Take another medium-sized bowl or deep plate and add the flour and nutritional yeast. Stir and dip each asparagus fry in the dry mixture until coated.

5. Repeat this for all the fries. Then transfer the asparagus fries to the baking sheet.

6. Bake for 20-25 minutes, or until golden brown.

7. Serve the fries with a vegan dip sauce, and enjoy!

8. Alternatively, store the asparagus in the fridge, using an airtight container, and consume within 4 days. Store in the freezer for a maximum of 30 days and thaw at room temperature. Use a toaster oven or pan to reheat the quiche.

Tip: Add chili flakes, garlic powder, or white pepper for another taste.

18. Egg Casserole

Nutrition Information
(per serving)
- Calories: 498 kcal
- Net Carbs: 4.7 g.
- Fat: 44.1 g.
- Protein: 19.6 g.
- Fiber: 7 g.
- Sugar: 2.5 g.

INGREDIENTS:
- 6 large organic eggs
- ½ cup cheddar cheese (shredded)
- ½ cup heavy whipping cream
- ½ small yellow onion (diced)
- 1 tsp. Dijon mustard
- ½ tsp. dried oregano
- Optional: 2 tbsp. grass-fed butter
- 2 medium Hass avocados (peeled, pitted, and sliced)
- Sea salt and ground black pepper to taste

Total number of ingredients: 10

METHOD:

1. Preheat oven to 350°F / 175°C.

2. Take a large bowl and crack in the eggs. Add the cheddar cheese, whipping cream, diced onions, mustard, oregano, and salt and pepper to taste.

3. Use a whisk to incorporate these ingredients into a smooth mixture.

4. Pour the contents of the bowl into a casserole dish and, if desired, top it with the optional butter.

5. Bake the casserole in the oven for 25-30 minutes, until the butter has melted and the top layer of cheese is brown.

6. Take the casserole dish out of the oven and allow it to cool for a few minutes.

7. Serve each portion with ⅓ of the avocado slices and enjoy!

8. Alternatively, store the casserole in the fridge, using an airtight container and consume within 3 days. Store in the freezer for a maximum of 30 days and thaw at room temperature. Use a microwave, toaster oven, or pan to reheat the casserole.

Tip: Substitute goat cheese for the cheddar cheese. Add freshly chopped parsley, thyme, and/or sweet paprika powder for another flavor!

19. Special Zucchini Lasagna

Nutrition Information
(per serving)
- Calories: 202 kcal
- Net Carbs: 5.4 g.
- Fat: 15.2 g.
- Protein: 10.1 g.
- Fiber: 3.4 g.
- Sugar: 2.8 g.

INGREDIENTS:

Walnut Sauce:
- 1 cup walnuts (ground)
- 1 cup simple marinara sauce (page 35)
- ¼ cup sundried tomatoes (chopped)
- Optional: pinch of salt

Tofu Ricotta:
- 1 14-oz. package firm tofu (drained)
- ¼ cup fresh basil
- 1 tbsp. lemon juice
- 4 tbsp. nutritional yeast
- 2 small garlic cloves (minced)
- 1½ tbsp. olive oil
- Salt and pepper to taste

Lasagna:
- 2 zucchinis (thinly sliced)
- 2 cups simple marinara sauce (page 35)
- Salt and pepper to taste

Total number of ingredients: 16

METHOD:

1. Preheat the oven to 375°F / 180°C.
2. Add the walnut sauce ingredients to a blender. Blend the ingredients into an almost completely smooth mixture.
3. Transfer the mixture to a medium-sized bowl and set it aside.
4. Clean the blender container and then add all tofu ricotta ingredients. Blend until smooth.
5. Take a pan and add 2 cups of simple marinara sauce. Cover the sauce with the zucchini slices and top these with ⅓ of the tofu ricotta. Pour half of the walnut sauce on top.
6. Make another layer, starting with zucchini slices, then tofu ricotta, and then the remaining walnut sauce.
7. Finish the lasagna with a layer of zucchini slices and tofu ricotta. Top the dish with some additional salt and pepper to taste.
8. Transfer the lasagna to the oven and bake for 30-35 minutes.
9. Allow the lasagna to cool down before serving and enjoy!
10. Alternatively, store the lasagna in the fridge, using an airtight container, and consume within 4 days. Store in the freezer for a maximum of 30 days and thaw at room temperature. Use a microwave, toaster oven, or pan to reheat the lasagna.

Tip: Incorporate vegan or dairy cheese in this lasagna. The final layer can also be topped with extra cheese or crushed walnuts.

20. Tofu Stir-Fry with Almond Bread

Serves: 4 | Prep Time: ~30 min |

Nutrition Information
(per serving)
- Calories: 380 kcal
- Net Carbs: 6.2 g.
- Fat: 30.6 g.
- Protein: 17.7 g.
- Fiber: 14.2 g.
- Sugar: 3.3 g.

INGREDIENTS:
Almond Bread:
- 1 cup almond flour (unflavored)
- 4 tbsp. psyllium husk
- 2 flax eggs (page 34)
- 1½ tsp. baking powder
- 1½ cups hot water
- 1½ tbsp. apple cider vinegar
- Pinch of salt

Tofu Scramble:
- 1 tbsp. coconut oil
- 1 shallot (finely minced)
- 2 tsp. turmeric powder
- 1 tbsp. sweet paprika powder
- 2 tbsp. nutritional yeast
- Black pepper to taste
- Sea salt to taste
- 2 cups of kale (chopped)
- ½ cup of cherry tomatoes (halved)
- 1 8-oz. pack extra firm tofu

Topping:
- 1 medium Hass avocado (peeled, pitted, and sliced)
- Optional: 2 tbsp. roasted sesame seeds
- Optional: ½ cup spring onions (chopped)

Total number of ingredients: 20

METHOD:
1. Preheat the oven to 400°F / 200°C, and line a baking tray with parchment paper.
2. Mix all the dry bread ingredients in a medium-sized bowl.
3. Use a whisk and your hands to incorporate the flax eggs, water, and apple cider vinegar with the dry ingredients. A firm dough should be formed. Add more water if necessary.
4. Divide the dough into 4 flattened buns.
5. Transfer the buns to the baking tray and put this in the oven.
6. Bake the flat almond bread for about 40 minutes. Flip the buns after 20 minutes.
7. Take the baking tray out of the oven and allow the buns to cool off.
8. Chop the tofu into tiny cubes and set it aside.
9. Take a medium-sized skillet, put it over medium heat, and add the coconut oil.
10. Stir in the minced shallot, turmeric powder, paprika powder, yeast, pepper, and salt to taste.
11. Add the chopped kale and heat the ingredients for about 2 minutes while stirring.
12. Stir in the chopped tofu cubes and top the ingredients in the skillet with the halved cherry tomatoes. Stir the tofu scramble for a minute before turning off the heat.
13. Take the almond buns and top them with the tofu scramble.
14. Add the avocado slices and, if desired, garnish with the optional spring onions.
15. Sprinkle the optional sesame seeds over the toppings, serve, and enjoy!
16. Alternatively, store the bread and tofu scramble, separated, in the fridge. Use airtight containers and consume within 4 days. Store in the freezer for a maximum of 30 days and thaw at room temperature. Use a microwave, toaster oven, or pan to reheat the scramble.

Tip: Top the almond bread with some pumpkin seeds or incorporate these into the dough.

1. No-Carb Cereal Bars

Nutrition Information
(per serving)
- Calories: 223 kcal
- Net Carbs: 2.4 g.
- Fat: 20.3 g.
- Protein: 7.2 g.
- Fiber: 3 g.
- Sugar: 0.8 g.

INGREDIENTS:

- 1 cup pumpkin seeds
- 1 cup sunflower seeds
- 1 cup almonds
- 1 cup hazelnuts (chopped)
- 1 flax egg (page 34)
- ¼ cup almond butter
- ¼ cup cocoa butter
- 1 tsp. stevia powder
- Ground cinnamon to taste

Total number of ingredients: 9

METHOD:

1. Preheat oven to 350°F / 175°C, and line a shallow baking dish with parchment paper.
2. Transfer all the listed ingredients to a blender or food processor. Blend it into a chunky mixture.
3. Transfer the mixture onto the baking dish and spread it out evenly into a flat chunk on the parchment paper.
4. Bake this chunk for about 15 minutes.
5. Take the baking dish out of the oven and let cool down for about 10 minutes.
6. Cut the chunk into the desired number of bars while it's still a bit warm.
7. Enjoy right away or store in the fridge, using an airtight container, and consume within 6 days. Store each bar separately in the freezer, using Ziploc bags, for a maximum of 90 days. Thaw the bars at room temperature.

SNACKS

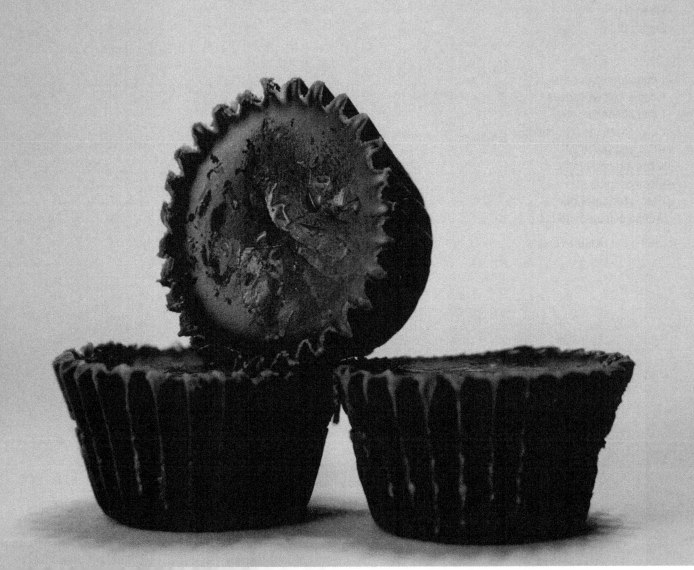

2. Nutty Chocolate Bombs

Serves: 12 cups | Prep Time: ~60 min |

Nutrition Information
(per serving)
- Calories: 253 kcal
- Net Carbs: 2.6 g.
- Fat: 24.7 g.
- Protein: 4.8 g.
- Fiber: 2.2 g.
- Sugar: 1.4 g.

INGREDIENTS:

Nut Butter Bottom:
- ½ cup coconut oil
- ½ cup peanut butter
- ½ cup almonds (chopped)
- ½ cup hazelnuts (chopped)
- ½ tbsp. pumpkin spice

Chocolate Top:
- ¼ cup cocoa butter
- 2 tbsp. cocoa powder
- ½ tsp. stevia powder

Total number of ingredients: 8

METHOD:

1. Line a muffin tray with muffin liners.

2. Put the coconut oil and peanut butter in a small bowl. Heat the bowl in the microwave for 10 seconds, or until the oil and butter have melted. Make sure it doesn't get too hot.

3. Transfer the melted ingredients and the remaining nut butter bottom ingredients to a food processor or blender. Blend everything into a chunky mix.

4. Transfer 1 tablespoon of the mixture from the blender into each muffin liner.

5. Repeat this process until the blender container is empty, making sure that all 12 muffin liners are evenly filled.

6. Put the muffin tray in the freezer for about 30 minutes, until the bottom layers are firm.

7. Warm up the cocoa butter in a small saucepan over low heat until it's completely melted.

8. Stir in the cocoa powder and stevia powder. Make sure the chocolate top ingredients are well incorporated.

9. Take the muffin tray out of the freezer and divide the chocolate top mixture over the muffins. Use a teaspoon and make sure the chocolate top mixture gets evenly distributed.

10. Put the muffin tray with the covered cups back in the freezer for another 30 minutes, until the nutty chocolate bombs are firm and ready to serve.

11. Enjoy right away or store in the fridge, using an airtight container, and consume within 6 days. Store the bombs in the freezer, using a Ziploc bag, for a maximum of 90 days. Thaw the bombs at room temperature.

3. No-Bake Hazelnut Chocolate Bars

Serves: 16 bars | Prep Time: ~60 min |

Nutrition Information
(per serving)
- Calories: 185 kcal
- Net Carbs: 1.8 g.
- Fat: 18 g.
- Protein: 3.4 g.
- Fiber: 2.4 g.
- Sugar: 0.8 g.

INGREDIENTS:
- ½ cup coconut oil
- 2 cups hazelnuts
- ¼ cup almonds
- ¼ cup walnuts
- 1 tbsp. pure vanilla extract
- 1 tsp. stevia powder
- ¼ cup cocoa powder

Total number of ingredients: 7

METHOD:

1. Line a shallow baking dish with parchment paper.

2. Transfer all the listed ingredients to a food processor or blender. Blend the ingredients into a chunky mixture.

3. Transfer the mixture onto the baking dish and spread it out evenly into a flat chunk.

4. Cover the baking dish and put it in the freezer for 45 minutes, until the chunk is firm.

5. Take the baking dish out the freezer, cut up the chunk into the desired number of bars, and store, or serve and share.

6. Enjoy right away or store in the fridge, using an airtight container and consume within 6 days. Store each bar separately in the freezer, using Ziploc bags, for a maximum of 90 days. Thaw the bars at room temperature.

4. Coconut Chocolate Balls

Serves: 24 balls | Prep Time: ~60 min |

Nutrition Information
(per serving)
- Calories: 210 kcal
- Net Carbs: 2 g.
- Fat: 20.8 g.
- Protein: 3.5 g.
- Fiber: 2.5 g.
- Sugar: 0.9 g.

INGREDIENTS:
- ½ cup coconut oil
- 1 cup almond butter
- 1 cup macadamia nuts
- ½ cup cocoa butter
- 1 cup shredded coconut flakes (unsweetened)
- 6 tbsp. cocoa powder
- 1 tbsp. vanilla extract
- 1 tsp. stevia powder

Total number of ingredients: 8

METHOD:

1. Transfer all the listed ingredients—except the shredded coconut flakes—to a food processor or blender. Blend the ingredients into a smooth mixture.

2. Line a baking tray with parchment paper to prevent the balls from sticking to the plate.

3. Scoop out a tablespoon of the chocolate and coconut mixture and roll it into a firm ball by using your hands.

4. Repeat the same for the other 23 balls. Coat each ball with the shredded coconut flakes and then transfer them to the baking tray.

5. Put the baking tray in the freezer for 45 minutes, until all balls are solid.

6. Take the baking dish out the freezer and store the coconut balls, or, serve them right away. Share the coconut chocolate balls with others and enjoy!

7. Alternatively, store the chocolate balls in the fridge, using an airtight container and consume within 6 days. Store the balls in the freezer, using Ziploc bags, for a maximum of 90 days and thaw the at room temperature.

5. Raspberry Cheesecake Fudge

Serves: 12 | Prep Time: ~60 min |

Nutrition Information
(per serving)
- Calories: 178 kcal
- Net Carbs: 4.7 g.
- Fat: 12.7 g.
- Protein: 10.9 g.
- Fiber: 1.9 g.
- Sugar: 2.1 g.

INGREDIENTS:
- ½ cup coconut cream
- 1 cup raw cashews (unsalted)
- ½ cup macadamia nuts (unsalted)
- ½ cup vegan protein powder (vanilla flavor)
- 2 tsp. nutritional yeast
- 2 tbsp. freeze-dried raspberry powder

Total number of ingredients: 6

METHOD:
1. Line a deep baking dish with parchment paper.
2. Transfer all the listed ingredients to a food processor or blender. Blend the ingredients into a smooth mixture.
3. Transfer the mixture onto the deep baking dish and spread it out into an even layer.
4. Put the baking dish in the freezer for 45 minutes, until the fudge chunk is firm.
5. Take the baking dish out the freezer, cut the chunk into the desired number of fudge servings, and enjoy right away!
6. Alternatively, store the fudge in the fridge, using an airtight container, and consume within 6 days. Store in the freezer for a maximum of 90 days and thaw at room temperature.

6. Blueberry Lemon Choco Cups

Serves: 12 | Prep Time: ~60 min |

Nutrition Information
(per serving)
- Calories: 178 kcal
- Net Carbs: 1.5 g.
- Fat: 18.7 g.
- Protein: 0.8 g.
- Fiber: 1.1 g.
- Sugar: 0.4 g.

INGREDIENTS:
- ½ cup cocoa butter
- ½ cup coconut oil
- ¼ cup cocoa powder
- 2 tbsp. organic lemon zest
- ¼ cup fresh lemon juice
- ½ tsp. stevia powder
- 20 blueberries

Total number of ingredients: 7

METHOD:

1. Put the cocoa butter and coconut oil in a medium bowl. Heat this bowl in the microwave for 10 seconds, until the butter and oil have melted. Make sure it doesn't get too hot.

2. Take the bowl out of the microwave and mix in all the remaining ingredients. Make sure everything is well incorporated.

3. Line a muffin tray with muffin liners.

4. Scoop the soft mixture out of the bowl with a tablespoon into the muffin liners. If the mixture isn't soft enough to be transferred, heat it again in the microwave for 10 seconds.

5. Fill all the muffin liners evenly, 1 tablespoon at a time.

6. Refrigerate the cups for 45 minutes, until the choco cups are firm. Take the cups out, serve and enjoy!

7. Alternatively, store the blueberry lemon cups in the fridge, using an airtight container, and consume within 6 days. Store in the freezer for a maximum of 90 days and thaw at room temperature.

7. Creamy Coconut Vanilla Cups

Nutrition Information
(per serving)
- Calories: 139 kcal
- Net Carbs: 1.6 g.
- Fat: 13.5 g.
- Protein: 2.6 g.
- Fiber: 1.4 g.
- Sugar: 0.7 g.

INGREDIENTS:
- ½ cup almond butter
- ¼ cup coconut cream
- ½ cup shredded coconut flakes (unsweetened)
- ¼ cup coconut oil
- 1 tbsp. vanilla extract
- 1 tsp. stevia powder
- Optional: 1 tsp. ground cinnamon

Total number of ingredients: 7

METHOD:
1. Put the almond butter, coconut cream, and coconut oil in a small saucepan. Heat the pan over medium-low heat while whisking the ingredients until molten and mixed together.

2. Take the pan off the heat and set it aside. Let the mixture cool down.

3. Pour the mixture into a medium-sized bowl and mix in the remaining ingredients.

4. Line a muffin tray with muffin liners.

5. Scoop the soft mixture out of the bowl with a tablespoon into the muffin liners.

6. Fill all the muffin liners evenly, 1 tablespoon at a time.

7. Refrigerate the cups for 45 minutes, until the coconut cups are firm.

8. Serve and enjoy, or, store the creamy coconut vanilla cups in the fridge, using an airtight container, and consume within 6 days. Store in the freezer for a maximum of 90 days and thaw at room temperature.

8. Peanut Butter Power Bars

Serves: 16 | Prep Time: ~60 min |

Nutrition Information
(per serving)
- Calories: 178 kcal
- Net Carbs: 2 g.
- Fat: 16.8 g.
- Protein: 4.6 g.
- Fiber: 1.4 g.
- Sugar: 1.4 g.

INGREDIENTS:
- ¼ cup almond butter
- ½ cup peanut butter
- ½ cup coconut oil
- ¼ cup sunflower seeds
- ¼ cup walnuts (chopped)
- ¼ cup hemp seeds
- 1 tbsp. vanilla extract
- 1 tsp. stevia powder

Total number of ingredients: 8

METHOD:

1. Put the almond butter, peanut butter, and coconut oil in a small saucepan. Heat the saucepan over medium-low heat and whisk the ingredients until everything is molten and fully incorporated.

2. Take the pan off the heat and set the mixture aside to cool down.

3. Line a baking dish with parchment paper.

4. Pour the contents of the saucepan into a medium-sized bowl and mix in the remaining ingredients.

5. Transfer the mixture onto the baking dish and spread it out into an even layer.

6. Put the baking dish in the freezer for 45 minutes, until the chunk is firm.

7. Take the baking dish out the freezer and cut the chunk into the desired number of bars.

8. Enjoy right away or store in the fridge, using an airtight container, and consume within 6 days. Store each bar separately in the freezer, using Ziploc bags, for a maximum of 90 days. Thaw the bars at room temperature.

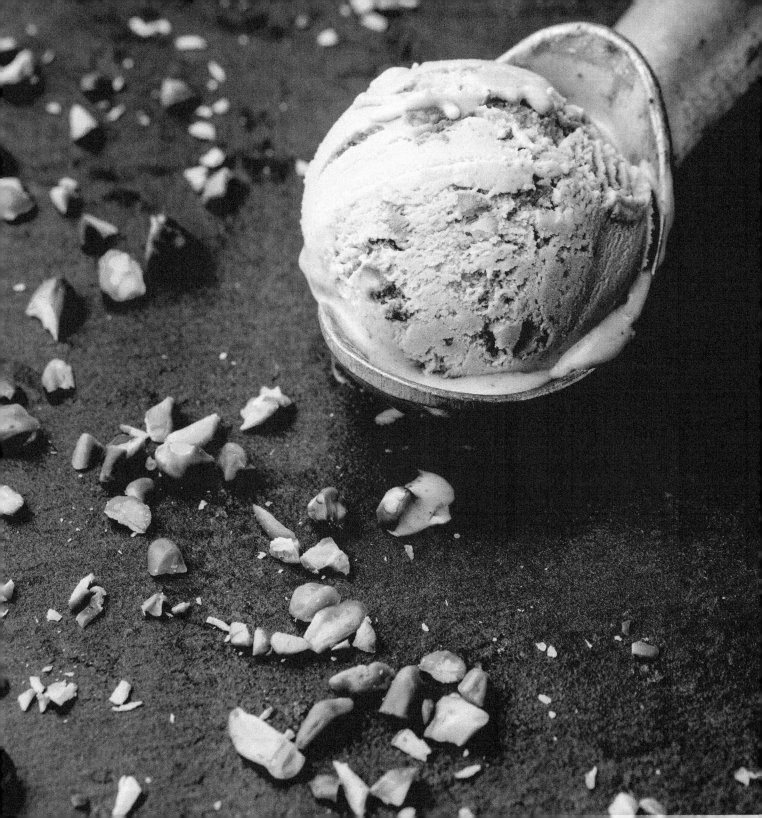

9. Low-Carb Pistachio Gelato

Serves: 16 | Prep Time: ~60 min |

Nutrition Information
(per serving)
- Calories: 320 kcal
- Net. Carbs: 6.5 g.
- Fat: 29.95 g.
- Protein: 5.8 g.
- Fiber: 2 g.
- Sugar: 2.85 g.

INGREDIENTS:
- 2 cups raw cashews (unsalted)
- 4 cups full-fat coconut milk
- ½ cup coconut oil
- 1½ cups pistachios (unsalted and shelled)
- 1 tsp. almond extract
- 2 tsp. tapioca starch
- ½ tsp. salt
- 1 tsp. stevia powder

Total number of ingredients: 8

METHOD:

1. Cover the cashews in a small bowl filled with water, and let sit for 4 to 6 hours. Rinse and drain the cashews after soaking. Make sure no water is left.

2. Add 1 cup of pistachios to a blender or food processor, or, alternatively, use a coffee grinder; blend or grind the pistachios into a fine powder.

3. Keep or add the pistachio powder into the blender or food processor. Add the soaked nuts and the other ingredients except the remaining pistachios. Blend the ingredients into a smooth mixture.

4. Transfer the mixture to an ice cream maker and make the gelato according to the appliance's instructions. Alternatively, mix the leftover pistachios into half of the ice cream mixture and freeze it for about 4 hours. Store the other half in the fridge for this time.

5. Further blend both mixtures in the blender or food processor into the desired gelato consistency.

6. Transfer the gelato to an airtight container and put it in the freezer for about 3 hours.

7. Let the gelato thaw for 15 minutes before serving. Enjoy!

8. The pistachio gelato can be stored, using an airtight container, for a maximum of 12 months. Thaw for about 5 minutes before serving.

10. Dark Chocolate Mint Cups

Nutrition Information
(per serving)
- Calories: 151 kcal
- Net Carbs: 1.3 g.
- Fat: 15 g.
- Protein: 2.3 g.
- Fiber: 1.5 g.
- Sugar: 0.4 g.

INGREDIENTS:
- ½ cup cocoa butter
- ½ cup almond butter
- ¼ cup coconut oil
- ¼ cup cocoa powder (unsweetened)
- 1 tsp. mint extract
- 1 tbsp. vanilla extract
- 1 tsp. stevia powder

Total number of ingredients: 7

METHOD:

1. Put the cocoa butter, almond butter, and coconut oil in a small saucepan. Heat the saucepan over medium-low heat. Incorporate the ingredients using a whisk, add the cocoa powder, and whisk again until all ingredients are fully incorporated.

2. Take the saucepan off the heat and set it aside to cool down.

3. Line a baking dish with parchment paper.

4. Pour the mixture from the saucepan into a medium-sized bowl and mix in all the remaining ingredients. Make sure all ingredients are fully incorporated.

5. Transfer a tablespoon of the mixture from the bowl into each muffin liner.

6. Repeat this process until the bowl is empty, making sure that all 16 muffin liners are evenly filled.

7. Refrigerate the cups for 45 minutes, until the coconut cups are firm.

8. Take the cups out of the freezer, serve, and enjoy right away.

9. Alternatively, store the chocolate mint cups in the fridge, using an airtight container, and consume within 6 days. Store in the freezer for a maximum of 90 days and thaw at room temperature.

11. Toasted Cashews with Nut Flakes

Serves: 3 | Prep Time: ~20 min |

Nutrition Information
(per serving)
- Calories: 338 kcal
- Net Carbs: 11 g.
- Fat: 27.9 g.
- Protein: 10.3 g.
- Fiber: 2.2 g.
- Sugar: 3.7 g.

INGREDIENTS:

- 1 cup cashews (unsalted)
- ¼ cup toasted coconut flakes
- 4 tbsp. almond flakes
- 1 tbsp. liquid monk sweetener
- ½ tbsp. cinnamon
- 4 tbsp. water
- ½ tsp. vanilla extract
- Sea salt to taste

Total number of ingredients: 8

METHOD:

1. Put a medium-sized frying pan or skillet over medium heat.
2. Add the liquid monk sweetener, cinnamon, salt, water, and vanilla extract. Stir the ingredients until everything is combined.
3. Then add the cashew nuts while constantly stirring. Make sure to coat all the nuts evenly in the liquid mixture.
4. Keep stirring while the liquid starts to crystalize on the nuts.
5. Transfer the toasted cashews to a plate and allow them to cool down.
6. Add the toasted coconut flakes and almond flakes, and then enjoy right away.
7. Alternatively, store the nuts in the fridge, using an airtight container, and consume within 10 days.

Note: Raw coconut flakes can be toasted in the oven at 325°F / 160°C for 5-10 minutes.

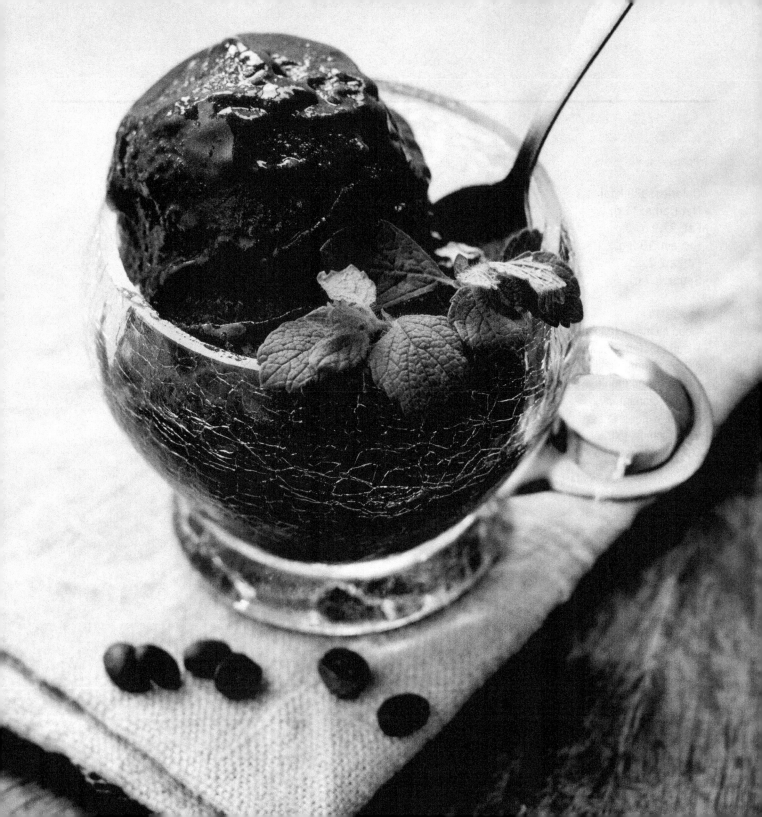

12. Choco Chip Ice-Cream with Mint 🥛 or 🌿

Serves: 8 | Prep Time: ~60 min |

Nutrition Information
(per serving)
- Calories: 275 kcal
- Net Carbs: 4 g.
- Fat: 27.2 g.
- Protein: 3.7 g.
- Fiber: 1.2 g.
- Sugar: 1.4 g.

INGREDIENTS:

- 2 cups heavy whipping cream (use coconut cream for vegan ice cream)
- ½ tbsp. agar-agar
- 1 ½ tbsp. water
- ¼ tsp. stevia powder (more depending on the desired sweetness)
- ½ scoop organic soy protein (chocolate flavor)
- ½ tbsp. instant coffee powder
- 1 tsp. salt
- 3 tsp. vanilla extract (more depending on desired taste)
- 4 tsp. peppermint oil (more depending on desired taste)
- 6 tbsp. dark chocolate (85% cocoa or higher, use chunks or crush a chocolate bar)
- Handful fresh mint leaves (chopped)

Total number of ingredients: 11

METHOD:

1. Put the heavy whipping cream in a large bowl and freeze it for at least 20 minutes.

2. Take out the cream and use a whisk to whip it for up to 10 minutes. Transfer the bowl back to the freezer.

3. In a medium-sized pan, add the agar-agar and water. Stir until the agar-agar has dissolved in the water, and then blend in the stevia powder.

4. Stir in the instant coffee powder and salt. Put the pan over medium heat. Stir constantly while heating the mixture, and make sure that no lumps remain.

5. Take the pan off the heat and stir in the protein powder. Set the mixture aside to cool down.

6. Take the whipped cream and add the vanilla extract and peppermint oil. Use more of both for a stronger taste.

7. Add the vegan gelatin mixture from the pan to the cream. Incorporate both mixtures by using a whisk or an electric mixer. This process is best done by working with multiple batches.

8. Taste the mixture and add more stevia, vanilla, and/or peppermint, depending on desired taste.

9. Freeze the mixture for 15 minutes. Stir it and freeze for another 10 minutes.

10. Top the ice cream with the dark chocolate chunks and freeze for at least 2 hours.

11. Allow to defrost 5 minutes before serving. Top with some additional dark chocolate, chopped mint, and enjoy!

12. The ice cream can be stored in an airtight container for a maximum of 12 months. Thaw for about 5 minutes before serving.

13. Chocolate & Yogurt Ice Cream

Serves: 1 | Prep Time: ~60 min |

Nutrition Information
(per serving)
- Calories: 355 kcal
- Net Carbs: 8.7 g.
- Fat: 17.9 g.
- Protein: 36.7 g.
- Fiber: 6.5 g.
- Sugar: 3.7 g.

INGREDIENTS:
- ⅔ cup low-fat Greek yogurt
- 1 scoop organic soy protein (vanilla or chocolate flavor)
- 1 tbsp. cocoa powder (unsweetened)
- 1 cup unsweetened almond milk
- 4-6 drops stevia sweetener (or low-carb maple syrup)
- 4 tbsp. almonds (crushed, alternatively use almond flakes)

Total number of ingredients: 6

METHOD:
1. Take a medium-sized bowl and add the Greek yogurt, protein powder, cocoa powder, almond milk, and stevia sweetener. Use a whisk to combine the ingredients together.

2. Put the bowl into the freezer for an hour.

3. Stir the ice cream and put it back in the freezer for 30 minutes. Repeat this step.

4. After 2 hours, the ice cream is ready for consumption. Allow it to soften for 5 minutes, top it with the crushed almonds, serve, and enjoy!

5. The ice cream can be stored, using an airtight container, for a maximum of 12 months. Thaw for about 5 minutes before serving.

Note: This ice cream can also be prepared using an ice cream maker.

14. Crispy Cheese Snacks 🥛 🥚

Serves: 4 | Prep Time: ~10 min |

Nutrition Information
(per serving)
- Calories: 248 kcal
- Net Carbs: 3.6 g.
- Fat: 15.9 g.
- Protein: 21.6 g.
- Fiber: 7.2 g.
- Sugar: 0.6 g.

INGREDIENTS:
- 2 medium organic eggs
- ½ cup cheddar cheese (shredded)
- ¼ cup parmesan cheese (shredded)
- ½ cup almond flour
- 1 8-oz. package tempeh
- 1 tsp. paprika powder
- Sea salt and black pepper to taste

Total number of ingredients: 8

METHOD:

1. Preheat the oven to 400°F / 200°C, and line a baking tray with parchment paper.

2. Take a medium-sized bowl and mix the eggs, cheeses, flour, and spices in it by using a spoon. Make sure that no lumps remain.

3. Divide the mixture in 8 even portions.

4. Cut the tempeh into 8 chunks.

5. Cover each piece of tempeh with a piece of the cheese mixture.

6. Transfer the snacks to the baking tray. Bake them in the oven for 12 minutes, until golden brown.

7. Allow the snacks to cool down before serving and enjoy!

8. Alternatively, store the cheese snacks in the fridge in an airtight container, and consume within 5 days. Store in the freezer for a maximum of 60 days and thaw at room temperature. Use a toaster oven to reheat the cheese snacks after freezing so they don't get soggy.

Conclusion

I would like to thank you for purchasing this book and taking the time to read it. I hope that it has been helpful to you!

The Ketogenic Vegetarian diet is very beneficial for your health and stamina. The combination of these two diets is one of the best you can find for your physical well-being and mental performance. Commit to it and you will reap the benefits!

Did you like this book? Then don't forget to leave a review on Amazon!

This way other readers can get inspired too.

Love,

Lydia

Sources

1   https://www.ncbi.nlm.nih.gov/pmc/articles/PMC5409832/
2   https://www.ncbi.nlm.nih.gov/pmc/articles/PMC5452247/
3   http://www.jlr.org/content/30/11/1727.abstract
4   https://www.nature.com/articles/0802369
5   https://www.ncbi.nlm.nih.gov/pmc/articles/PMC3945587/
6   https://en.oxforddictionaries.com/definition/vegetarian
7   https://www.ncbi.nlm.nih.gov/pubmed/9416027
8   https://www.livestrong.com/article/267249-amino-acid-supplements-for-women/https://www.ncbi.nlm.nih.gov/pmc/articles/PMC4935284/
9   https://www.ncbi.nlm.nih.gov/pmc/articles/PMC4935284/
10   https://www.nutrition.org.uk/nutritionscience/nutrients-food-and-ingredients/protein.html?limit=1&start=2
11   *Dietetics Manual by Jean Lederer*
12   https://www.aafp.org/afp/2009/0101/p43.html
13   https://academic.oup.com/ajcn/article/101/6/1317S/4564491
14   https://www.ncbi.nlm.nih.gov/pmc/articles/PMC3449675/
15   http://www.who.int/nutrition/publications/nutrientrequirements/WHO_TRS_935/en
16   http://www.dummies.com/health/nutrition/what-are-simple-carbohydrates-complex-carbohydrates-and-dietary-fiber
17   http://www.diabetes.org/food-and-fitness/food/what-can-i-eat/understanding-carbohydrates/glycemic-index-and-diabetes.html
18   https://www.cambridge.org/core/services/aop-cambridge-core/content/view/AF44097B0E9C4FF9BD44F1D55CD353D6/S0007114514002931a.pdf/does_cooking_with_vegetable_oils_increase_the_risk_of_chronic_diseases_a_systematic_review.pdf
     https://www.sciencedirect.com/science/article/pii/S0278691510004941?via%3Dihub
19   https://www.ncbi.nlm.nih.gov/pubmed/29511019
20   https://www.ncbi.nlm.nih.gov/pmc/articles/PMC4365303/
21   https://www.ncbi.nlm.nih.gov/pmc/articles/PMC4892314/
22   https://www.ncbi.nlm.nih.gov/pmc/articles/PMC5646809/
     https://www.ncbi.nlm.nih.gov/pmc/articles/PMC2974200/
23   https://www.ncbi.nlm.nih.gov/pubmed/12442909
24   https://www.ncbi.nlm.nih.gov/pmc/articles/PMC5611753/
     https://www.gbhealthwatch.com/Science-Omega3-Omega6.php
25   https://www.joslin.org/info/how_does_fiber_affect_blood_glucose_levels.html
26   fiberfacts.org/fibers-count-calories-carbohydrates
27   'A ketogenic diet as a potential novel therapeutic intervention in amyotrophic lateral sclerosis' by Zhao et al
     'Ketogenic diet protects dopaminergic neurons against 6-OHDA neurotoxicity via up-regulating glutathione in a rat model of Parkinson's disease' by Cheng et al
     'The ketogenic diet: metabolic influences on brain excitability and epilepsy' by Lutas & Yellen

Made in the USA
Monee, IL
05 March 2020